THE **PALEO PROJECT**

The 21st Century Guide to Looking Leaner,
Getting Stronger and Living Longer

DR. MARC BUBBS

ND, CSCS

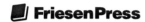

Suite 300 - 990 Fort St
Victoria, BC, Canada, V8V 3K2
www.friesenpress.com

ISBN
978-1-4602-5202-4 (Hardcover)
978-1-4602-5203-1 (Paperback)
978-1-4602-5204-8 (eBook)

1. Health & Fitness, Weight Loss

Distributed to the trade by The Ingram Book Company

CONTENTS

ACKNOWLEDGEMENTS

I would like to thank all the people who have ignited my passion for health, exercise and wellness. Without the revolutionary work of Dr. Linus Pauling and Dr. Udo Erasmus, which truly opened my eyes to the concept of promoting health rather than treating disease, this journey would undoubtedly never have begun. To my naturopathic professors and mentors, I am eternally grateful for your guidance and support: Dr. Paul Saunders, Dr. David Leischeid, Dr. Kim Whitaker, Dr. Natasha Turner, Dr. Erin Wiley, and Dr. Megan Walker. Thank you as well to my mentors in the world of athletics: Clance Laylor, Sam Gibbs, and Chris Broadhurst. I am indebted to the work and readings of many great Paleo researchers and experts: Dr. Boyd Eaton, Dr. Loren Cordain, Dr. Art De Vany, Dr. Deborah Gordon, Robb Wolf, Nora Gedgadaus, Chris Kresser, and Mark Sisson. Your wisdom and foresight has helped millions of people improve their health. Lastly, and most importantly to my wife Carly and my daughter Zadie for inspiring me on this journey, as well my family and close friends. This would not have been possible without your love and support.

INTRODUCTION

Welcome to *The Paleo Project*. In the next ten chapters I am going to take you on a journey that will empower you to upgrade your mental and physical performance, emotional wellbeing, and overall health.

As a naturopathic doctor and strength coach, I have always had the fundamental belief that *what you eat* and *how you move* are the cornerstones of health.

In fact, it all starts in your brain. World-renowned neuroscientist Dr. Daniel Wolpert believes there is only one reason why you have a brain. Can you guess what it is? *Movement.*

Your brain is designed to assess incoming information so you can produce adaptive and complex movement in order to survive. It's no wonder that movement is so intricately connected to your mood, your digestive system, your immune system, your hormonal systems and everything in between. The better you move and the more you move, the better your quality and length of life. Years ago, doctors scoffed at this idea. Today, science is backing it up.

Let's take this a step further. Do you know the most important marker of your general health and life expectancy? (Don't feel bad, most doctors aren't aware either.) Lean muscle! As a percentage of your bodyweight, your lean muscle mass is the single most important marker of your health. For example, compare a slightly overweight person with someone who looks to be of average weight. If the overweight person has more muscle mass than the average-weight person, the latest research shows the former is more likely to be healthier and to live longer!

This is an amazing finding because it reframes the conversation *away* from "weight loss" and shifts the focus towards "strength gain." Losing excess weight is good for you, but gaining muscle is even better for you! The new mantra making waves in the online community, "strong is the new skinny," should be taken to heart. Regardless of whether you are trying to improve your body composition, upgrade your health or reach a new level of performance, strength is the foundation.

We are all athletes. We are all born to crawl, squat, bend, run, jump, smile and laugh along the way. These qualities are effortless and natural when we are children, yet somehow we lose touch with them as we get older. Ultimately, we all need to learn to reconnect with our "inner athlete" (it doesn't matter if you've never played a sport in your life or if you were an all-star athlete; challenges are present at both ends of the spectrum.)

It's my belief that movement, strength and a balanced diet are the basis to improve your health, to fit into your new pair of jeans or to reach a new personal best time.

Unfortunately, our lifestyle today is more sedentary and the way we eat has dramatically changed. The sad truth is that if you simply go with the flow—consuming processed foods, simple sugars, and unhealthy fats that are so prevalent, leading a hectic lifestyle, struggling to find fulfilment in your work or making time to move and play—you'll get swept away by the current of weight gain and poor mental, emotional and physical health.

We live in a world where it's increasingly difficult to maintain *your* ideal bodyweight, feel happy and vibrant, and fight off pain and chronic diseases. The World Health Organization (WHO) predicts that by the year 2050 *one-third* of the global population will develop type-2 diabetes. The WHO also predicts by that same year *one-third* of the planet will suffer from anxiety or depression. Does this seem acceptable? Why are we struggling to eat, live and be happy?

Examining our ancestral roots is the key to our success in the future. We need to reconnect with how we've evolved from our hunter-gatherer past into the complex humans we are today. This is where the "Paleo" portion of my book title fits into the equation.

For those who are unfamiliar with the Palaeolithic diet, it is also known as the "caveman" diet, hunter-gatherer diet or ancestral diet. It consists of a diet centred on foods that were staples of our hunter-gatherer ancestors millennia ago and therefore, presumably, more appropriate to our genetic make-up. The diet emphasizes the most nutrient dense foods—quality-raised animal protein, healthy fats, abundant vegetables and fruits, nuts and seeds—while limiting processed foods, simple sugars and alcohol.

Like most diets, people thought the Paleo diet was just another fad. Nothing could be further from the truth. New studies are continually being published in the scientific literature highlighting the many health benefits of a Paleo dietary approach: improved blood sugar control, reduced risk of diabetes, cancer and cardiovascular disease (ironically, with the consumption of *more* meat, not less), fewer auto-immune conditions and weight loss, among others.

In this book, I'll walk you through my Modern Paleo approach. A Modern Paleo diet uses the Paleo philosophy as the foundation on which to build your own personalized *best* diet. The strictest interpretation of the Paleo diet calls for the complete removal of all grains, legumes and dairy. However, current nutritional research suggests that some of these foods—rice, lentils, yogurt, etc.—do not exert the detrimental effects originally believed by hard-line Paleo followers and could actually support *better* health in some people.

I will use the term "Modern Paleo" throughout the book to imply that I am taking into account the latest advances in nutritional research, rather than simply adhering to a dietary protocol that attempts to mimic what a "caveman" would have eaten. For example, plain yogurt is a fantastic food to increase your protein intake and get a beneficial dose of health-promoting probiotics. Brown rice is a wonderful *hypoallergenic* (meaning it does not typically cause food allergies) carb option that improves the balance of good gut bacteria, provides a rich dose of vitamins and minerals, and supports optimal performance and recovery.

These foods are typically *not* allowed under the strictest of Paleo rules, but for many they provide great benefit. In the Modern Paleo approach, the Paleo diet is the platform from which you can build the best diet for *you*!

In fact, in clinical practice I try to avoid using labels for dietary strategies. Whether it's a Pritikin diet, the South Beach diet, a vegetarian diet, the Zone diet, or even the Paleo diet, using labels to define how you eat confines you. I believe your diet should emphasize the foods *you* need to be vibrant and healthy, correct natural deficiencies and work in harmony with your genetics, type of work, intensity of training, etc.

You may be wondering why I chose to call my book *The Paleo Project* if I don't believe people should label their diets. The truth is that everyone needs a starting point. There is no better reference point or standard for what a modern diet should include than an ancestral or Paleo approach to eating.

In Section I of this book, you'll learn how to use a Modern Paleo dietary approach to build the foundation of your own *best* diet. A Paleo approach naturally eliminates the most harmful foods—simple sugars, trans fats, processed foods, glutens, etc.—from the diet, while emphasizing foods that are important in achieving your best health—quality proteins, healthy fats, abundant alkalinizing vegetables and fruits, and foods naturally rich in fibre and electrolytes.

This doesn't mean you need to convert to a 100% Paleo lifestyle. The *Paleo Project* is about discovering how adding more Paleo-based meals to your day or to your life may have a profound impact on how you feel, think and perform (at work and in the gym). In this book, you'll uncover just how profoundly an ancestral approach to eating, naturally more in tune with your genetics, dramatically affects key areas of your body (digestion, immunity, inflammation, blood-sugar control and stress response).

Nutrition is so critical to improving health, losing weight and ramping up performance that I've put it at the base of my *Paleo Project Pyramid* (Figure A), a framework for helping you build your best body from the inside out. The *Paleo Project Pyramid* shows the importance of solidifying the most basic aspects of health—diet, digestion, immunity, inflammation, hormone balance—so that you can *achieve* and *sustain* better health, your best body and your performance goals.

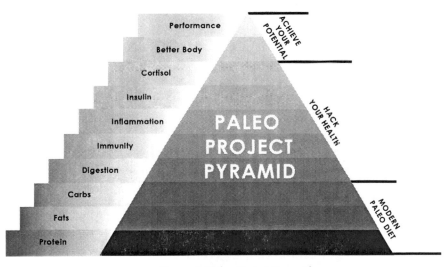

Figure A. Paleo Project Pyramid

You may be wondering about the "project" aspect of this book. The "project" in *The Paleo Project* is the transformational journey you are about to embark on (both mind and body, as the two are intimately connected). I'll provide you with the roadmap to assess how efficiently your body is functioning, effectively *hacking your health* to uncover imbalances or key deficiencies that may be holding you back from achieving better health, a better body or better performance.

If you are not sure what hacking your health means, it's the use of functional testing to assess how efficiently or optimally your body is functioning. The traditional medical system lab tests were designed to uncover *disease*. While this is important in fighting off illness, the current medical model is biased toward treating disease rather than promoting health. Hacking your health is intended to improve your health by uncovering imbalances and areas that need support *before* they become dysfunctional.

Think of it as examining the squeaky wheel on your car. It's best to do this before the wheels actually fall off the proverbial cart! Just as you would ensure your business is running efficiently, your job or department at work is highly productive, or your investments are yielding the greatest gains, you should ensure you have the same mindset concerning your health.

If you wait for things to go wrong and *then* attempt to correct them, it's much more difficult to fix the problem. You wouldn't wait until your business was about to go bankrupt to make a change, so why do the same for your health?

In Section II of *The Paleo Project*, I'll guide you through a series of self-assessments so you can identify areas of imbalance, deficiency or weakness. If you find areas that need improvement, you'll learn about the latest functional lab tests designed to hack your health and identify the cause of your imbalance or dysfunction. From there, I'll provide you with dietary and supplemental strategies to bring your dysfunction back into balance.

Supplements are a hot topic these days. It seems that more and more people are carrying around bottles of pills, powders and gels in their quest for optimal health, weight loss and better performance. I believe your *diet* should provide you with everything you need to be happy, healthy and achieve optimal performance. That is why each chapter in Section II (Hacking Your Health) implements food-based strategies to correct and support health in the long term.

There is a time and a place for supplements. The definition of a *supplement* is a substance taken to remedy a deficiency in a person's diet. The supplement protocols given in this book are designed to do just that—correct deficiencies in your digestive, immune, inflammatory or hormonal function. The more severe the dysfunction is, the more comprehensive the supplement strategy.

I typically recommend clients take supplements for four to eight weeks, then assess and re-evaluate their progress. If you've applied the correct remedy, you'll likely no longer need to supplement. Food sources should then fill the gap left by the supplements to maintain your health or performance in the long term.

In general, supplements should be used when you have an increased need for nutrients (e.g., during intense training or times of stress), if you have an inherent deficiency (e.g., low iron or B12) or if you have an imbalance or dysfunction in a particular area of the body. Otherwise, what you eat, how you move and your lifestyle are far more powerful influencers of your health than simply popping a pill.

As you move through each chapter, you'll be moving up the *Paleo Project Pyramid* one rung at a time. For example, if you pass your self-assessment for digestive function in Section II, you'll move on to hacking your immune system in the next chapter. If everything is on point with immunity, you'll continue to Chapter 6 (Inflammation), the next rung on the *Paleo Project Pyramid*. If at any point, you uncover an imbalance or deficiency, you'll follow the appropriate *Action Plan* to restore optimal function.

Finally, in Section III of *The Paleo Project* you are going to reconnect to your inner athlete. Whether you are an absolute beginner in terms of exercise, or an experienced gym-goer striving to achieve *better movement* will make it easier to achieve your goals and improve your health.

I'll shift your focus away from working out not just to *look* better but to *live* better. By reframing the conversation toward movement and striving to achieve higher quality and more functional movement, you will become more athletic, improve your fitness, increase your capacity to burn fat and build muscle, and best of all you'll have the ultimate foundation for better health and quality of life.

In Section III, you get to choose your own adventure. If fat loss and transforming your body is your primary target, Chapter 9 will provide you with the tools to achieve your goals. If upgrading your performance and achieving a new personal best is your priority, Chapter 10 will lay the framework to realize those goals.

In short, I'll be asking you to choose weight loss/better body or performance as your ultimate benchmark, not both. Why is that? While you can achieve both, if you are looking to make the *most significant gains*, keep your eyes on a single goal.

Aiming for two goals at different ends of the spectrum commonly leads to sub-optimal results in both. For example, being 6% body-fat (versus 8%) will not help your performance when deadlifting your maximum weight, running your fastest 10k, or completing a difficult CrossFit WOD (workout of the day). On the contrary, being able to perform a fast cycling time trial or perform heavy Olympic lifts does not necessarily translate to six-pack abs or a beach body.

While there is some crossover, if you can keep "performance" and "body composition" (weight loss, "getting leaner," etc.) separate in your mind, you'll achieve your goals more quickly. Once your first goal has been reached, you can move on to the next one!

The Paleo Project reflects the fundamental principles of how I view health, wellness and performance, and how I treat clients in clinical practice. I have experienced firsthand how health and performance suffer if your nutrition and body systems are dysfunctional. In my late teens I suffered major digestive and immune problems that derailed my senior athletic season in high school. After failing to see progress after visiting the "best" doctors and specialists, I visited a naturopath in Toronto who changed my diet, corrected my digestive ailments and supported my immune system. My improvement was rapid, profound and got me back on the playing field in no time.

A project is defined as a collaborative enterprise. There is an entire community out there already eating more in tune with our ancestral roots and redefining the notion of body image and health. My hope is that the *Paleo Project* can not only help you in your journey to better health and performance but also connect you more closely with communities (both online and in your hometown) that prioritize movement and eating in tune with nature as essential aspects of life.

Make YOU your *project* for this year. To complete *The Paleo Project*, work your way through the *Paleo Project Pyramid* until you achieve your final goals in Section III. For some, this journey will be quick, for others it may take some time. I hope this book provides a spark to ignite your quest to building a stronger, leaner, healthier YOU!

Enjoy the journey!

SECTION I

The Modern Paleo Diet

"Let food be thy medicine; let medicine be thy food."
~Hippocrates

Did you know that 85% of all chronic diseases—high blood pressure, high cholesterol, heart disease, diabetes and many cancers—are caused by diet, exercise and lifestyle factors? That even elite and professional athletes often have deficiencies in their diet? And that the best way to lose weight is via a better diet, not more exercise? Whether your goal is to improve your health, your body composition or take your performance in the gym or at the office to the next level, look no further than your plate.

A poor diet leads to an inadequate intake of essential proteins, fats, vitamins and minerals that are necessary for health and wellness. Incredibly, the average person is deficient in almost ten important nutrients. This shortened supply has ripple effects throughout the body.

A poor diet can disrupt your digestion (leading to gas, bloating and abdominal discomfort), compromise your immunity (leading to more colds and flu), cause systemic inflammation (resulting in joint pain and poor health), and hormonal imbalances. All these factors contribute to weight gain, increased risk of chronic disease and poor performance.

The *Paleo Project Pyramid* is the platform for rebuilding your body from the ground up and the foundation is your nutrition. What you eat has the greatest impact on your health, performance and all systems in your body. That's why it's at the base of the pyramid. If your diet is poor or inadequate, the function of key systems—digestion, immunity, inflammation and hormone production—will also be poor or inadequate. This may compromise your ability to build muscle, lose weight or achieve your performance potential. Build a solid nutritional platform and your quest for better body composition, better health and better performance will be accelerated.

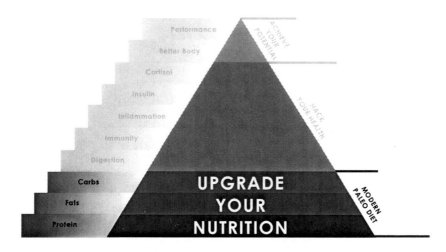

Figure B. The Paleo Project Pyramid—Section I

In Section I of *The Paleo Project* (Figure B), I'll discuss the fundamentals of nutrition—proteins, fats, and carbohydrates—and show you how to develop the best diet for you. If you're new to the Paleo world, you'll learn fantastic insights into how adding more Paleo-type meals can improve your health and performance. If you're already a Paleo-eater, you'll learn the benefits of a Modern Paleo approach and how customizing your Paleo diet helps fill in the gaps, correct deficiencies and individualize your eating to promote better health and performance.

You hear so much conflicting information in newspapers and magazines about fad diets and "the latest exotic supplement from the depths of the jungles" that it's difficult to decipher the real information from the junk. I'll expose many diet myths commonly seen in fad diets that steer you in the wrong direction and I'll discuss the latest research that will change your body. Do you eat enough protein? Do you eat the right kinds of fat? Are you eating too many carbs? Section I gives you the tools to answer these questions.

I'll also discuss the common pitfalls that sabotage your health, weight loss and progress in the gym. By identifying these common roadblocks, you can upgrade your diet and build a solid foundation for success.

At the end of each chapter, you will receive an *Action Plan* that will set the standard for building *your* best diet. As you move through the book, your dietary recommendations will continue to evolve, based on your current health, imbalances and overall goals and will ultimately take shape in Section III at the end of the book.

Take your first step to better health, a better body and better performance than you ever thought possible!

CHAPTER 1

PROTEIN—The Athlete's Power

Proteins are the building blocks of life: the bricks and mortar of your body. If you are training hard or working long hours (or both!), making sure you eat enough protein is critical for your performance, recovery and general health.

Proteins are essential for your body. They build:

- Red blood cells that provide oxygen to your cells

- Hormones that help build lean mass and burn body fat

- Immune cells that fight off bacteria and viruses

- Neurotransmitters that influence emotions and thought

- Muscle tissue to support exercise and general health

Your protein intake greatly influences how well you look, feel and perform. For performance, protein builds the critical lean muscle mass needed to run faster, jump higher and lift heavier objects. The athletic mantra *"bigger, faster, stronger"* would be impossible to achieve without adequate protein consumption.

Not everyone is training for performance. Many people simply want to stay active, lose weight, and feel vibrant and healthy. If your goal is to trim your waistline or improve your energy level, determining your optimal protein intake is very important. It helps you build muscle, burn body fat, improve mental focus, support positive mood and boost your immunity. There is no better way to increase your daily protein intake than to adopt a more Paleo-friendly diet.

I. BACK TO BASICS—PROTEINS 101

AMINO ACIDS

Regardless of whether you eat a chicken breast, salmon fillet or a handful of almonds, the proteins you consume are broken down in your gut to their simplest form: the individual amino acid. The human body contains 20 basic amino acids, which are the building blocks of proteins. They are made up of only four things: oxygen, hydrogen, carbon and nitrogen elements. Figure 1.1 shows you the basic structure of an amino acid.

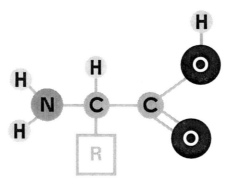

Figure 1.1. Basic Structure of an Amino Acid

Essential Amino Acids

Your body is capable of producing 11 of the 20 basic amino acids internally with its own cellular machinery. These amino acids are classified as *non-essential*. The remaining nine are called *essential amino acids* because your body cannot produce them and must obtain them from your diet. The nine essential amino acids include phenylalanine, valine, tryptophan, threonine, isoleucine, methionine, histidine, leucine and lysine. Animal proteins are richest in essential amino acids.

Conditionally Essential Amino Acids

Under stressful circumstances a sub-group of non-essential amino acids are required in much greater quantities by your body. They are referred to as *conditionally essential amino acids*, because even though your body can make them, under stressful conditions they are needed in much greater quantities. The *conditionally essential amino acids* include arginine, cysteine, glutamine, glycine, ornithine, proline and tyrosine.

Who needs these conditionally essential amino acids? Take an athlete, for example, who is training intensely. He would require greater amounts of glutamine to cope with added stress on the body and immune system. Similarly, a desk worker logging long hours and exercising multiple times per week may also have a higher need, based on the increased mental and physical stress.

Branched-Chain Amino Acids

Leucine, isoleucine and valine are a group of three essential amino acids that are classified as the *branched-chain amino acids* (BCAAs). BCAAs make up about one-third of your total muscle protein pool, making them key players in your nutritional arsenal. In particular, the branch-chain amino acid leucine is the all-star of the group for its exceptional ability to increase lean muscle, improve recovery and enhance performance.[1, 2, 3]

Leucine also supports fat loss by influencing your blood sugar hormone insulin and supporting the conversion of the amino acid alanine into glucose to be used as an instant energy source.[3, 4] This makes BCAAs very effective in supporting weight loss. Animal source proteins such as red meat, chicken, fish and dairy products are the richest sources of leucine and BCAAs.

The Final Protein Product

When your body is trying to build a certain protein, it needs to have all the amino acids present. If even one essential amino acid is absent, the desired protein cannot be built. This is known as a *rate-limiting amino acid*. It's also the key reason why an optimal intake of dietary essential amino acids is crucial in achieving your weight loss, performance and health goals.

To appreciate the complexity of various proteins, consider that insulin is made up of a 51 amino acid sequence, the satiety hormone leptin is comprised of 167 amino acids, and growth hormone (GH) is 191 amino acids. Your body is able to produce over 100,000 different proteins from only 20 different amino acid building blocks— simply amazing!

Protein Digestion

After consuming a protein-rich meal, your stomach has the important task of breaking down the proteins into smaller tri-peptides (three amino acid chains), di-peptides (two amino acid chains), and individual amino acids. It does so by producing gastric juices made up of hydrochloric acid (HCl) and the enzyme pepsin. These gastric juices are very acidic so your stomach secretes a mucous layer to protect the inner lining from damage.

As the partially digested proteins pass through your stomach into the small intestine, your pancreas joins in to help, secreting enzymes that further breakdown the amino acids so they can be absorbed more easily into your bloodstream.

Once the amino acids have made it into your bloodstream, they can be used in four different ways:

- To build new tissues (muscles, hormones, immune cells, neurotransmitters, etc.)

- To be oxidized or burned directly for energy

- To be converted to glucose (a process called gluconeogenesis)

- To be converted into fat.

Proteins are not entirely clean-burning fuels. The diagram in Figure 1.2 illustrates how protein metabolism produces ammonia and urea waste by-products that must be excreted by the kidneys. This places a mild burden on your kidneys, so remember to drink plenty of water to support optimal clearance of urea. A simple blood test can tell if your urea levels are high.

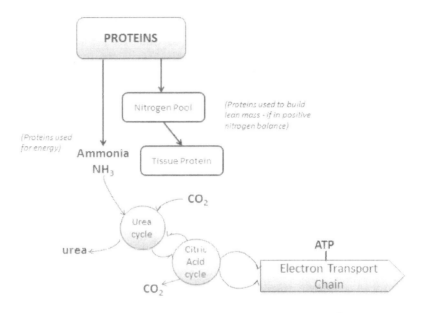

Fig 1.2. The By-Products of Protein Metabolism.[5]

II. THE BIG DEBATE—THE BEST SOURCES OF PROTEIN

This question is one of the most common questions asked by my clients in clinical practice. Should I avoid red meat? Is fish the best option? Should I be eating more vegetarian proteins? New fad diets come out every year promising to revolutionize the future of nutrition but the truth is that scientific research is uncovering that eating the way our grandparents and great grandparents did (and all the way back to our Paleolithic ancestors) is more likely to benefit you. It includes grass-fed beef, wild game meats, ocean fresh fish, naturally raised chicken, omega-3 rich eggs, and fruits and veggies from nutrient rich soils, that dramatically improve the nutrient profile of the food you eat.

Many scientific assessment methods are used to rank the quality of a protein source. Today, the two most commonly used methods to assess protein quality are *biological value* (BV) and *protein digestibility amino acid score* (PDCAAS).

The BV method measures the amount of nitrogen consumed versus the amount absorbed, with values taken from both humans and animals. The PDCAAS assessment tool compares the first limiting amino acid of a protein source versus a reference pattern, theoretically giving you a better assessment of the amino acid profile for each protein source.

Which one should you use? Well, the answer is both. Consider both BV and PDCAAS when evaluating the quality of a protein because no one measurement can provide all the necessary information.[6, 7] In this section I'll walk you through the most common sources of protein. When comparing protein types consider that the optimal value of PDCAAS is 1.0, the highest biological value of protein food sources is 100, and supplemental sources approximately 160.

FOOD SOURCES OF PROTEINS
Animal Proteins

When it comes to quality protein, animal sources are truly "king of the jungle." They contain *all* essential and conditionally essential amino acids and have the highest protein absorption rate of all foods. They are also the richest source of BCAAs and creatine (a high energy protein) both of which are critically important in building lean muscle mass, burning fat, improving performance and upgrading general health.

What most people don't realize is that animal protein is extremely *nutrient dense*. It contains the highest concentrations of essential vitamins and minerals, nutrients, essential amino acids and essential fats. Meat is incredibly good for you; you just need to find quality-raised meat.

However, there can be some drawbacks with animal protein consumption, such as possible increased exposure to antibiotics and heavy metals. To limit these disadvantages, select meats from local and sustainable farms that raise their animals naturally, with respect for the animals and the environment. The table in Figure 1.3 outlines the various animal protein sources.

Source	PDCAAS	BV	DISADVANTAGES
Cow Milk	1	91	Allergies to lactose and/or casein
Eggs (whole egg)	1	100	Common food allergy
Casein (e.g. cottage cheese)	0.8 - 0.9	77	Allergies, Indigestible
Meat (e.g. steak)	0.8 - 0.9	80	Use of antibiotics and hormones
Poultry (e.g. chicken)	0.8 - 0.9	79	Use of antibiotics and hormones
Fish (e.g. salmon)	0.8 - 0.9	76	Heavy metals

Figure 1.3. Comparison of Animal Protein Sources

Vegetable Proteins

Vegetable proteins are considered inferior to animal proteins because they are typically deficient in one essential amino acid. Vegetarian proteins are also inferior because they are absorbed at only 70% efficiency compared to animal sources. If you follow a diet devoid of animal protein, you may be short of the full complement of essential amino acids necessary to achieve a better body, better performance and better health.

To correct for this deficiency, though, vegetarians and vegans should obtain a *mix* of vegetable protein sources at every meal. In general, grains are deficient in the amino acid lysine and beans are low in methionine. By combining two of the following three food groups—beans and pulses, grains, and nuts/seeds—you should be able to achieve sufficient levels of all the essential amino acids.

If you are vegan/vegetarian and beans are your primary source of protein, consider the following. First, beans are high in the sugar raffinose that causes gas, bloating and abdominal discomfort in most individuals. Next, beans contain trypsin-inhibitors that impair the digestive enzyme trypsin that is needed to break down proteins. Thirdly, beans contain significant levels of phytates and oxalates, which are anti-nutrients that block the absorption of important minerals such as zinc, magnesium, calcium and iron. Finally, beans contain lectins that are intestinal irritants, causing damage to the lining of the intestinal tract.

In a strict Paleo diet, all beans and legumes are off limits. However, if you are vegan or vegetarian your best bet is to limit your bean consumption (or eliminate it altogether) and opt for lentils instead. Red, green, and yellow lentils are easier to digest and typically contain greater levels of protein than beans. They can also be a nice addition to a Modern Paleo approach, as lentils are a very nutrient-dense food and well digested by most people.

Source	PDCAAS	BV	DISADVANTAGES
Soy	1.00	74	Mild extrogenic effect contains phytic acid and trypsin inhibitors
Beans (e.g. lima beans)	0.60	66	Contains phytates, lectins and trypsin inhibitors
Lentils	0.52	45	High-carb content
Corn	0.42	60	Allergic food for some people
Nuts (e.g. peanuts)	0.52	55	Allergic food for some people

Figure 1.4. Comparison of Vegetarian Protein Sources

PEANUT BUTTER AND TOXINS

If peanut butter is your number one choice for a vegetarian protein, don't buy the cheap stuff! Why? Peanuts contain aflatoxin, a potent natural mould or mycotoxin that is one of the most carcinogenic compounds on earth. It grows commonly in the soils of peanut fields and is extremely detrimental to your health and athletic performance. Always choose organic sources of peanut butter.

SUPPLEMENT SOURCES OF PROTEINS

If you are looking to improve your health, gain lean muscle or maintain high productivity at work, optimizing your protein intake is an absolute must. Don't short change yourself in the protein department. Supplemental sources of protein are ideal to use as a breakfast option (to increase the protein content), before or after bouts of exercise or as a healthy snack. They are absorbed much faster than food sources of protein, which has a dramatic impact on your ability to build muscle and recover from exercise. In Figure 1.5, I describe the most common forms of protein supplements. I'll discuss the pros and cons for each type below so you can determine the best option for you.

Source	PDCAAS	BV	DISADVANTAGES
Whey Isolate	1	160	Allergies to lactose and/or casein
Whey Hydrosylates	1	160	Common food allergy
Whey Concentrate	1	104	Allergies, poor digestion
Casein	1	77	Allergies, poor digestion
Soy Protein	1	74	Use of antibiotics and hormones
Rice Protein	0.47	83	Arsenic levels
Pea Protein	0.69	65	Low BV
Hemp Protein	0.46	60	Low BV

Figure 1.5. Comparison of Supplemental Protein Sources

Whey Proteins

Whey protein is at the head of the class when it comes to supplemental proteins. It is derived from the cheese-making process, when milk proteins are divided into portions of curds (casein protein) and whey. Approximately 80% of the protein derived from milk is in the casein form, while the remaining 20% is whey protein. Cheese manufacturers actually used to throw out the whey portion during the cheese-making process, thinking it was simply a waste product. Today, it is one of the most popular and profitable supplements in the world!

You can consider several different forms of whey protein: whey protein isolate, whey concentrate and whey protein hydrosylates.

Whey Protein Isolate

Whey protein isolate has the highest possible biological value (approximately 160) and PDCAAS scores (equal to 1.0 or 100%) of any food or supplement. This makes it the undisputed #1 *choice* for supplemental protein.

What makes it so effective? Whey protein isolate contains a high concentration of leucine, the branched-chain amino acid that stimulates the genetic pathways (mTOR) that trigger muscle protein synthesis.[1, 2] Leucine is the spark that tells your DNA to build lean muscle. Whey isolate is also one of the richest sources of glutathione, your body's most potent antioxidant, liver support and detoxifier.[8] It also supports healthy cardiovascular function by lowering elevated blood pressure in as little as six weeks![9]

Whey isolate is ideal to consume before, during or after exercise because it is rapidly absorbed into your bloodstream (within an hour). It is also a good option to consume first thing in the morning when your body is in *negative* nitrogen balance after a long night's sleep.

Despite all these benefits, whey isolate is not for everyone. If you suffer from dairy allergies, you may need to cut it out of your diet. Although it contains less than 1% lactose—the disaccharide sugar found in milk—it might still cause gas and bloating in some people. Symptoms of a whey allergy include fatigue, sinus congestion, post-nasal drip, frequent colds and flu, brain fog and poor recovery from training. (If this sounds like you, I cover this in more detail in Chapter 4—Digestion.)

Whey Protein Concentrate
Whey protein concentrate is the cheapest and most widespread type of whey protein. It typically has greater concentrations of vitamins, minerals and immune boosting nutrients, especially if you purchase grass-fed whey protein concentrate. However, whey concentrate has less protein (less than 80%) compared to whey isolate (greater than 90%) and higher lactose concentration, making it difficult to digest for those with dairy allergies. If you experience gas, bloating or cramping, you should discontinue use. Whey protein concentrate is still a highly absorbable and effective protein, with a PDCAAS score of 1.00 and a biological value of 104.

Whey Protein Hydrosylates

Whey protein *hydrosylates* are a more easily digestible form of whey protein. They are traditionally used in hospital settings with infants or elderly patients who have compromised digestive function. Whey hydrosylates are essentially pre-digested into smaller peptides compared to whey isolate or concentrate, which means they can reach peak levels in the bloodstream much faster.[10] (Pure pharmaceutical grade amino acids are absorbed fastest.[11])

If you cannot tolerate dairy or whey isolate due to allergies, give whey hydrosylates a try. You may be able to tolerate it due to its pre-digested processing. It is fantastic for building muscle and shedding body fat. The major drawback is that it tastes very poor and does not blend well. To compensate, try adding a scoop of whey hydrosylates to one scoop of vegetarian protein (if you are sensitive to whey isolate) to make it more palatable. If you have no problems digesting whey, a combination of whey isolate and hydrosylate is best.

Casein Protein

During the cheese-making process, milk proteins are divided into portions of curds and whey; *curds* are the *casein* form of protein. Casein is often referred to as *milk protein* because approximately 80% of protein derived from milk is in the casein form (although milk does contain *both* casein and whey).

Casein is a more slowly absorbed protein and is a good choice to consume before bed due to its slow release throughout the night. It has a BV of 77 and has been shown to increase lean muscle mass and improve hypertrophy and body composition in conjunction with strength training.

Despite these benefits, supplementing with casein is a little redundant. If you can digest casein, you can likely digest dairy products, so you are better off having some cottage cheese (high in casein) or a glass of milk before bed to accomplish the same goal.

WHAT ABOUT MILK AFTER TRAINING?

Years ago, bodybuilders, strongman trainees and elite athletes would have chosen to drink milk after exercise to build lean mass and accelerate recovery. Today, the research shows not much has changed!

In multiple studies, milk was compared with soy protein or carbohydrate supplement post-training, and the results were not even close. Those people consuming milk post-workout had a much greater increase in strength, hypertrophy and were actually leaner than the other two groups. The results are clear. Drinking milk post-training makes you bigger, stronger and leaner! One cup of milk contains about 8g of protein, therefore men should aim for at least one litre (32g) and women at least 500ml (16g) after exercise.

IS MILK BETTER THAN WHEY ISOLATE?

The current research shows that milk performs just as well as the gold standard whey protein isolate as a post-exercise drink. This is a curious phenomenon for researchers because theoretically milk should NOT perform as well as whey isolate.

Why is this? Milk contains 80% casein protein, which is more slowly absorbed than whey isolate and considered an inferior choice after exercise. Next, milk contains far less muscle-building leucine than whey isolate, again suggesting it should be an inferior choice. Fortunately for milk drinkers, theory does not meet reality.

In spite of these factors, milk performs on par with whey isolate for promoting lean mass and strength gains. How is this possible? Expert researchers believe it's due to milk's ability to powerfully stimulate insulin release (an anabolic hormone), the variety of proteins found in milk (casein and whey), the presence of carbohydrates in milk (especially chocolate milk) and additional growth factors.[12]

IS SKIM MILK BETTER THAN FULL-FAT MILK?

If milk is a great post-training protein source, which kind is best: skim milk or whole milk? Recently, the journal *Medicine and Science in Sports and Exercise* shed some light on the question. They had 24 men and women engage in a strength-training program and divided them into three drinking groups: fat-free milk, whole milk and iso-caloric fat-free milk. The results showed that the whole-milk group had the greatest increase in muscle mass compared to the other two groups.[13] These results were consistent in both men and women. The scientific literature is quite clear. Whole milk is extremely effective for promoting gains in lean mass and strength after exercise.

ARE THERE ANY DISADVANTAGES WITH MILK?

Based on this evidence, why doesn't everyone supplement with milk, post-training? There are several key reasons why milk may not be the best option for you. If you suffer from food allergies to milk or dairy products due to either the lactose sugar or casein protein, you may experience symptoms such as gas, bloating, diarrhea, dark circles under the eyes, mucous build-up, frequent colds/flu and chronic nasal congestion.

In fact, milk and dairy consumption is a contentious topic in the Paleo world, with experts split on whether it's a healthy choice and should be included in a Paleo diet. In a Modern Paleo approach, milk can be consumed if you don't suffer from digestive or immune allergies.

It's important to note that you can be allergic to the lactose sugar or the casein protein or in some cases both! This inability to digest either the lactose sugar or casein protein can have ripple effects that disrupt your intestinal microflora, the balance of good and bad bacteria in your gut, and subsequently your health and performance.

Soy Protein

Soy protein is another *fast-acting* protein and the *only* true vegetarian protein source with a full complement of essential amino acids (yes, quinoa has a lot of protein for a carbohydrate, but in the protein weight class, it's still a lightweight!). Studies show that soy is almost as good as whey isolate and indeed better than whey concentrate at increasing lean muscle protein synthesis, strength and hypertrophy post-training.[7]

In Asia, fermented soy, called *tempeh*, is the predominant type of soy consumed. The fermentation process mitigates the negative effects of phytates in unfermented soy (e.g., tofu) and is highly beneficial for the gut. Soy protein has a biological value of 74 and PDCAAS score of approximately 0.91.

Over the last decade soy has become increasingly popular in protein bars and shakes, typically consumed in the *unfermented* form. But many problems exist with consuming too much unfermented soy. The major drawbacks include *raising estrogen* levels, high levels of *phytic acid* (a compound that inhibits calcium, magnesium, copper, iron, and zinc absorption), *trypsin inhibitors* (compounds that interfere with protein digestion) and *high aluminum levels* (a toxic heavy metal that inhibits cellular energy function). These concerns are serious. Limit yourself to two to three servings per week. (If you simply enjoy a splash of soymilk in your latte, I wouldn't worry about it.)

Rice and Pea Proteins

Rice and pea protein blends are vegetarian options gaining in popularity. With the increasing prevalence of dairy and whey allergies, rice and pea proteins offer a *hypo-allergenic* protein alternative, meaning most people will have no trouble digesting them and they won't irritate your immune system. They do not typically cause the fatigue, gas, bloating or brain fog and poor immunity associated with whey and dairy allergies.

Rice and pea proteins contain a full complement of essential amino acids but lower concentrations of BCAAs and creatine, making them inferior to whey for performance and recovery. They also have lower PDCAAS scores compared to whey isolate and concentrate. Rice and pea proteins should be used *only* if you cannot tolerate milk or whey protein, or if you are consuming multiple shakes per day.

In order to raise the bar and make rice and pea proteins on par with whey isolate, try adding BCAAs and creatine to your post-training shake to maximize lean muscle and recovery. It's not uncommon for people following a Paleo diet to have to use a vegetarian protein source after exercise due to allergies to whey protein and milk.

Hemp Protein

Hemp protein is another vegetarian protein source that has become increasingly popular with athletes seeking more vegetarian protein options. Although soy protein contains greater protein levels, hemp is easier to digest and does not contain trypsin-inhibitors. Hemp protein is also much less likely to cause allergic reactions than soy. The downside is that hemp protein has a poor biological value (60) and PDCAAS score (less than 0.5).

III. HOW THINGS GO WRONG

1) Not Enough Protein For Breakfast

The traditional North American breakfast includes cereal, toast, muesli, orange juice, muffins or pancakes. In other words carbs, carbs and more carbs! Breakfast is the most important meal of the day and if you don't get enough protein first thing in the morning, a lot of bad things can happen:

- Your focus will suffer due to low dopamine levels.

- You'll be constantly hungry due to low leptin levels.

- Your blood sugars will yo-yo up and down due to insulin spikes.

- You'll be craving carbs and stimulants to keep yourself going through the day.

It's no wonder 75% of the population is overweight. The current low-protein, low-fat, and high-carb breakfast is the perfect recipe for weight gain! A Paleo breakfast is the ideal solution to boost your morning protein intake.

2) Not Enough Protein in Your Smoothie

The growing trend of morning breakfast shakes or smoothies is a very healthy option. However, don't make the mistake of loading up the fruit and veggies and forgetting the most important ingredient! If you are struggling to lose weight or improve your health, then a high-carb, low-protein smoothie loaded with fruit is *not* your best bet. Your blood sugar and insulin hormone levels rise quickly with high-carb drinks (remember, liquids raise blood sugars much faster than real food) so if you are out of shape, wanting to shed a few pounds or trying to improve your health, you need to *add protein* to your smoothie to slow the release of sugars, keep your insulin levels in check and satiate your appetite throughout the day.

3) Not Enough Protein Around Exercise

A growing area of research in the world of sports nutrition is called *nutrient timing*, the concept that *when* you consume specific macronutrients (e.g., before, during or after training) can significantly alter your body composition, performance and recovery. This means that without even changing *what* you eat, simply changing *when* you eat your carbs, proteins and fats goes a long way to accelerating your progress.

Kicking off the research into nutrient timing, a study at the *University of Victoria* in Australia compared the difference between one group of athletes consuming a protein + creatine + carbohydrate shake for breakfast and dinner versus another group consuming exactly the same shake *before and after* exercise. The only difference between the two groups was *when* they had their shakes. The results were eye opening! The group consuming their shakes before and after training had significantly greater gains in lean muscle mass, strength (in the squat and bench press exercises), fast-twitch muscle fibres, as well as creatine and glycogen stores.[14] All of these benefits resulted from simply *timing* the nutrient intake around training bouts.

4) Too Many Sandwich Meats!

Meat gets a bad rap and sandwich meats are one of the main reasons. Sandwich meats are choked full of nitrites, which are extremely detrimental to your general health and in particular your digestive health. Nitrites are added to lunchmeats to act as a preservative and prevent against bacterial botulism infection. However, during cooking and processing these nitrites react to form potentially carcinogenic N-nitroso compounds.

Processed meats are typically classified as any meat that is smoked, cured, salted and filled with added preservatives. Studies show that people who eat large quantities of processed meats are at significantly greater risk of developing cardiovascular disease and colon cancer. So, skip the lunchmeats and eat *real* meat such as organic chicken, wild fish, grass-fed beef and wild game meats. Alternatively, you can try "nitrite-free" lunchmeats. These options will improve the quality of the protein in your diet.

IV. THE BENEFITS OF A HIGH PROTEIN DIET (AKA MODERN PALEO DIET)

Fat Loss and High Protein Diets

The Atkins Diet trend of the 1990s introduced the world to the benefits of a high protein diet for weight loss. Unfortunately, the diet's downfall was its lack of emphasis on fruit and vegetables and rumours that too much protein could be bad for your health. Doctors and nutritionists were commonly telling their patients to limit their meat and fat consumption if they wanted to stay healthy. Unfortunately, the current science doesn't back up those recommendations.

In 2007, the famous A-to-Z trial conducted by the prestigious *Journal of the American Medical Association* compared the effects of a high protein, high fat and low carbohydrate diet versus more traditional

Western-type diets (lower in protein and fat, higher in carbohydrates). Over 300 overweight and obese women participated in the study, and the results were very impressive. After 12 months on the high protein and high fat diet, the group that lost the most weight was the high protein diet group.[15] Countless other studies have confirmed these findings. It seems Dr. Atkins was on the right track!

Improve Satiety to Accelerate Fat Loss

How does more protein equal healthy weight loss? It all starts with your hunger and satiety signals. High protein diets improve your *satiety signal,* the hormones that tell your brain "I am full." With a better satiety signal, you can turn off the constant cravings for sugary snacks and avoid consuming food in excess.

Studies show that adopting a high protein diet leads to a decrease in your daily caloric intake, which translates into successful fat loss in the long term. How does this magic happen? Researchers have uncovered that increased leptin efficiency (leptin is the hormone that makes you feel full) is triggered by higher protein diets.[16] The better your leptin function is, the better your appetite control, and the slimmer your waistline.

Preserve Lean Muscle to Accelerate Fat Loss

High protein diets don't just make you feel full, they accomplish another important task—they preserve lean muscle mass. Maintaining your lean muscle mass is an absolute must for keeping your metabolism in top gear. Most fad diets cause you to lose precious lean muscle, muscle glycogen stores and water, which all weigh a lot more than fat! This translates into *more* weight loss but *not* fat loss. It's a classic fad-diet trick!

Simply adding more protein to your diet makes all the difference in the world for achieving your ideal body composition. A review study of over 1,000 people showed that high protein diets compared to standard protein intake were far superior in achieving weight loss, fat loss and preserving lean muscle mass.[17] If you can maintain your muscle, you will burn more fat and be on the way to better health and performance.

Belly-Fat and High Protein Diets

A high protein diet helps you to trim your belly-fat. If you would like to get leaner and find your six-pack abs, then adopting a high protein diet can make your dream a reality. A recent study demonstrated that adopting a high protein diet achieved the greatest abdominal fat loss, as well as weight loss, compared to a standard protein diet.[18] Waist circumference measurements are used in medical settings as a reliable indicator for evaluating your risk of developing chronic diseases; men should aim for *at least* less than 38 inches, while women should aim for *at least* less than 36 inches.

Improve Cholesterol and Cardiovascular Health

You may be wary of adopting a high protein diet because you've heard it may increase your cholesterol levels and increase your risk of heart disease. Once again, these myths are *not* backed up by science. The truth is that studies show that high protein (and high fat) diets elicit the greatest increase in good HDL cholesterol, a decrease in triglycerides (blood fats), and improvement in blood pressure compared to normal protein/low-fat diets.[14] The famous *OmniHeart* study by Harvard University supports the findings that high protein diets are far superior at lowering blood pressure than low protein, high carbohydrate diets.[19] To review the benefits of a high protein diet, check out Figure 1.6.

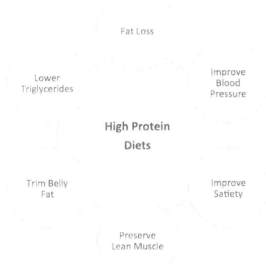

Fat Loss

Lower
Triglycerides

Improve
Blood
Pressure

High Protein

Diets

Trim Belly
Fat

Improve
Satiety

Preserve
Lean Muscle

Fig 1.6. Benefits of a High Protein Diet on Weight Loss and Overall Health

ARE THERE NEGATIVE SIDE EFFECTS TO TOO MUCH PROTEIN?

You often hear in the media that high protein diets can be dangerous for your health. This myth has persistently circulated on websites and in medical clinics. It is proposed that diets high in protein contribute to increased risk of cardiovascular disease, impaired kidney function and risk of osteoporosis. Do these claims have any merit?

A 2012 review in the *European Journal of Clinical Nutrition* analysed 74 clinical trials and noted that high protein diets significantly decreased blood pressure, blood lipids and adiposity.[20] (This is not conveyed by doctors or popular media). The Harvard School of Public Health supports these findings, recently releasing a study confirming that high protein intake does not increase the risk of coronary heart disease.[21] While popular myths may warn against high protein diets, the science supports high protein as actually health promoting.

Another common misconception is that high protein diets are dangerous to your kidneys. This claim is simply not supported by the latest research. Finally, high protein diets have been said to leach calcium out of your bones. A European study tested this hypothesis and concluded that high protein diets do not produce any changes in calcium excretion or absorption compared to placebo.[22]

V. THE PALEO PROJECT—PROTEIN SOLUTIONS

The science is clear. More protein equals quicker fat loss, better performance and superior overall health. Hit your optimal daily protein intake and start feeling the benefits for yourself. In order to maintain optimal cardiovascular health, robust immunity, strong muscles and bones, and positive mood, you need to consume the right amount of protein for you.

New research suggests the requirements are higher than you think. The *International Society of Sports Nutrition (ISSN)*, a group of world-renowned nutritionists, researchers, and doctors, recommends you aim for a total daily protein intake between 1.5 to 2.0g/kg bodyweight.[23] A Modern Paleo dietary approach is a great way to boost your protein consumption and achieve your optimal intake.

For example, a 200lb (91 kg) male should eat between 136 and 182 grams of protein daily. For a 140lb (64 kg) female, it would translate into 95 to 127g daily. What if you are not an athlete? (But remember, we are all athletes!) Start by aiming for the lower end of the recommended intake (1.5g/kg) to support better overall health.

Generally, men should consume a protein serving size equal to 1.5 to 2.0 *palm* sizes while women should aim for 1.0 to 1.5 palm sizes (a palm size in the width and thickness of the palm of your hand) at each mealtime.[24] This measurement translates into roughly a 30–40g protein serving for men and 20–30g serving for women.

What can you do if you are still short of your total suggested intake? Try increasing your protein portion sizes at meals, eating more frequent meals throughout the day or adding protein supplementation to help meet your total daily protein requirements. Liquid nutrition should always be prioritized around exercise, if possible.

Remember, a Modern Paleo diet emphasizes that *real food* sources of protein should make up the majority of your intake. One of the great benefits of a Paleo approach is that it forces you to prioritize *real food* rather than relying on bars, powders and pills. Most people don't realize that meat is the *most nutrient dense* food you can eat, containing an abundance of vitamins, minerals and essential nutrients! Be sure to include regular servings of the protein sources found in Figure 1.7.

Seafood	Wild Game	Meat	Other
Salmon	Bison	Grass-Fed Beef	Eggs (duck,
Mackerel	Venison	Chicken	chicken, goose)
Anchovies	Elk	Turkey	Dairy (yogurt)
Sardines	Rabbit	Pork	
Herring		Bacon	
Black Cod		Lamb	
Oysters		Goat	
Shrimp			
Mussels			
Lobster			
Clams			

Figure 1.7. High Quality Sources Of Protein

In order to achieve your ideal protein intake every day, you should have an action plan. Check out Figure 1.8 and the *Protein Solutions Action Plan* found there. Review the list of objectives and make sure you are incorporating all the action plan points to begin establishing the foundation of your health and performance.

```
┌─────────────────────────────────────────────────────────────┐
│                 PROTEIN SOLUTIONS ACTION PLAN                 │
├─────────────────────────────────────────────────────────────┤
```

1. Consume 1.5-2.0g/kg bodyweight of protein daily

- Men consume 1.5-2.0 'palms' of protein per meal; women 1.0-1.5 'palms'.

2. Consume a high protein breakfast

- Men 30-40g; Women 20-30g.

3. Eat a wide variety of animal protein sources

- If you are vegetarian tempeh should be your #1 protein option.

4. Include supplemental protein around exercise bouts

- Use whey protein isolate or milk post-training. If you have allergies to whey or dairy, use rice or pea protein.

Figure 1.8. Protein Solutions Action Plan

SAMPLE MENU

This section includes various meal and snack options for increasing your protein intake throughout the day. Simply adhere to the palm serving protocol outlined in the preceding section and feel free to substitute other sources of healthy animal protein. As you move through the next two chapters, you'll see more suggestions for fats and carbohydrate intake.

Breakfast Options

1. Eggs (3-6 for men; 2-4 for women)

2. Protein shake (30-40g for men; 20-30g for women)

3. Chicken breast (At least 1.5-2.0 palm sizes for men, 1.0-1.5 palm sizes for women)

4. Vegetarian option – full-fat plain yogurt (1.5 cups for women; 2.25 cups for men).

Snacks (AM)

- Walnuts (one handful, palm facing down)

- Full-fat yogurt (1.5 cups or 20g for women; 2.25 cups or 30g for men)

Lunch Options

1. Salmon fillet (at least 1.5-2.0 palm sizes for men, 1.0-1.5 palm sizes for women)

2. Grass-fed beef (at least 1.5-2.0 palm sizes for men, 1.0-1.5 palm sizes for women)

3. Turkey breast (at least 1.5-2.0 palm sizes for men, 1.0-1.5 palm sizes for women)

4. Vegetarian option — Tempeh (at least 1.5-2.0 palm sizes for men, 1.0-1.5 palm sizes for women)

Snacks (PM)

- Macadamia nuts (one handful, palm facing down)

- Full-fat plain yogurt (1.5 cups for women; 2.25 cups for men)

Dinner Options

1. Pork (at least 1.5-2.0 palm sizes for men, 1.0-1.5 palm sizes for women)

2. Black cod (at least 1.5-2.0 palm sizes for men, 1.0-1.5 palm sizes for women)

3. Bison (at least 1.5-2.0 palm sizes for men, 1.0-1.5 palm sizes for women)

4. Vegetarian option — Yellow lentils (at least 1.5-2.0 palm sizes for men, 1.0-1.5 palm sizes for women)

CHAPTER 2

FATS—The Athlete's Oil

You regularly hear the saying "You are what you eat" to emphasize that what you put into your mouth becomes the building blocks of your body. If you eat burgers and fries, your cells will be made up of burgers and fries. If you eat wild Alaskan salmon and broccoli, your cells will be made up of all the essential amino acids, fats, vitamins and minerals needed to build a healthy body.

Let's take this a step further. You are not only what *you* eat but you are also what your food ate! The foods chosen to feed animals have a tremendous impact on the quality of their meat and the nutrition humans get from consuming those animals. While farmers have known this for centuries, factory farming and the development of corporate farming has resulted in a major shift in the food chain. Animals are now being treated as commodities and, as a result, their health and nutritional quality is severely compromised.

This is not just a question of animal rights or the environment but a question of food quality. Did you know that the fats from grass-fed beef contain the same healthy omega-3 fats as heart-healthy salmon? That's right. However, eat grain-fed beef and the levels of beneficial omega-3s plummet; in its place are greater quantities of pro-inflammatory omega-6 fats. A major benefit of a Paleo dietary approach is its emphasis on naturally raised and wild game meats produced with respect for the animal, the farmer and the environment.

In Chapter 1, I discussed how proteins are the bricks and mortar of the body but in this chapter, I outline how fats are the *oil* that keeps your metabolic engine running smoothly. Essential for optimal athletic performance, weight loss and good health, fats play a critical role in establishing a solid nutritional foundation. By optimizing your intake of health-promoting fat, you can achieve quicker fat loss, improve your lifts in the gym, boost immunity, accelerate recovery and support hormonal balance.

I. BACK TO BASICS—FATS 101

STRUCTURE OF FATS

Fats do not like water. Each fatty acid molecule has one water-soluble or hydrophilic end, and one water insoluble or hydrophobic end (literally meaning *water fearing*). This characteristic gives fats many unique properties, allowing them to play a vital role in cellular communication. The ability of hormones and neurotransmitters—powerful chemical messengers in the body— to dock onto receptor sites on your cellular membranes requires optimal membrane fluidity and function.

All fats are classified as *acylglycerols* and are made up of two parts—one glycerol molecule and three fatty acids (acyl molecules). The glycerol molecule forms the backbone of the fat, which is attached to three fatty acid molecules. As soon as the glycerol backbone is removed, the fats are considered *free fatty acids* because they are free to travel through the bloodstream. Recall that fats hate water and free fatty acids are no different; they must be ferried through your bloodstream in a water taxi called a *carrier protein*, which shuttles them from one area of the body to another.

SATURATED FATS—NOT ALL BAD!

Saturated fatty acids (SFAs) are the most basic form of fatty acid and can be found in most foods containing fats or oils. They are abundant in fats that are "hard" at room temperature and doctors used to believe (many still do!) that all saturated fats are harmful to the body. While this is true for some saturated fats, it isn't the whole story. Over the past few decades, new research has shifted opinions and shown the many beneficial effects of good saturated fats.

a) Short-chain SFAs

Saturated fats can be classified as short-chain triglycerides (SCT), medium-chain triglycerides (MCT), or long-chain triglycerides (LCT). The SCTs are typically less than six carbons in length. They are absorbed directly by the gut (unlike most fats that must travel first to your liver to be processed), making them easy to digest and a source of instant energy. They also provide robust immune enhancing benefits. SCTs provide the foundation of optimal digestive function, a healthy balance of intestinal microflora and superior general health.

For example, butyric acid (4:0) is a powerful anti-microbial. It kills off harmful pathogens in your intestinal tract and promotes a healthy environment for good gut bacteria.[1] For this reason, real butter is terrific for your health—it's a great source of butyric acid! Coconut oil is another great source of butyric acid, as well as the good bacteria in your gut, which produces butyric acid when dietary fibre is fermented. If you're interested, Figure 2.1 shows the chemical structure of butyric acid. The diagram shows all the carbon, hydrogen and oxygen atoms.

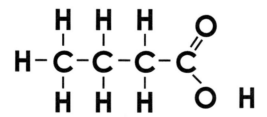

Figure 2.1. The Chemical Structure of Butyric Acid

b) Medium-chain SFAs

Medium-chain saturated fatty acids or medium-chain triglycerides (MCTs) are typically 8 to 12 carbon atoms in length. See Figure 2.2 for its"short-form" chemical structure. MCTs are the primary fuel for your enterocytes or gut cells, making them extremely important for digestive health. They also exert powerful anti-microbial effects on the body. For example, caprylic acid (8:0) is essential for fighting off the growth of harmful yeasts (i.e., candida albicans) and bacteria in your intestines.[1]

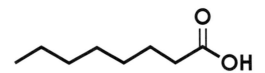

Figure 2.2. Chemical Structure of Caprylic Acid

MCTs are metabolized directly from the gut and used as an instant source of energy during exercise or to get you through your busy workday. They are highly fuel-efficient, providing you with nine calories/g of energy versus only four calories/g with carbs. This translates into *double* your fuel efficiency!

An added bonus for weight loss and overall health is that MCTs provide this energy without stimulating the release of insulin (your blood sugar hormone) the way carbohydrates do. Excessive insulin levels are a strong contributor to weight gain and the development of chronic diseases (more on insulin in Chapter 7). MCTs are a staple in the Modern Paleo diet and are found naturally in coconut oil, milk fats, butter, and ghee (clarified butter).

c) Long-chain SFAs

Long-chain saturated fatty acids or long-chain triglycerides (LCT) are associated with poor health and increased risk of heart disease. They are sticky in nature, leading to many of the negative health effects associated with consuming too many saturated fats. The negative effects include blood clots that clog arteries and lead to heart attacks or stroke.

However, LCTs do play an essential role in the body. They are used to construct cellular membranes and are vital for signalling and communication between cells of the body. LCTs are digested more slowly than SCTs and MCTs, and due to their size they must be first packaged up into chylomicrons (a carrier molecule) before travelling to your liver to be processed. Certain foods containing LCTs—namely, coconut oil, grass-fed butter and ghee—can be beneficial to the body, while deep-fried foods, processed foods and candies containing LCTs should be avoided.

AREN'T SATURATED FATS BAD?

You may be wondering: "Why does my doctor tell me to avoid saturated fats? Aren't they bad for me and cause heart disease?" Well, the work of world-renowned researcher Dr. Dariush Mozaffarian of Harvard University has shed new light on this old refrain and his findings may shock you. Recently, he summarized: "*Although the paradigm that saturated fat is a major cause of CHD [coronary heart disease] has become entrenched in the public and scientific consciousness over decades, modern nutritional evidence simply does not support a major effect of saturated fat on CHD risk.*"[2] Take it from the experts that not all saturated fats are bad.

In Figure 2.3 below, I have included a summary list of healthy saturated fats and their benefits.

Short-Chain Triglycerides	Increase 'good' bacteria
Medium-Chain Triglycerides	Fuel for energy production
Long-Chain Triglycerides	Build healthy cell membranes

Figure 2.3. Summary of Saturated Fats

UNSATURATED FATS—ESSENTIAL FOR HEALTH

The foundation for good health and athletic performance is a balanced intake of all fats—saturated, monounsaturated and polyunsaturated. Monounsaturated fats or MUFAs (commonly pronounced *moo-faas*) are classified as such due to the presence of one double bond within their chemical structure. Polyunsaturated fats or PUFAs (pronounced *poo-faas*) differ because they have two or more double bonds in their chemical structure and make up the third and final category of fats.

The presence of double bonds in MUFAs and PUFAs provides a kink in the fatty-acid chain, effectively changing its actions on the body. Structure equals function. Change the structure of the fat and you change the effect on the body. The double bond also has a mildly negative charge that allows it to spread apart in your cell membranes because like forces repel each other. These small but significant changes make your cell membranes more fluid and allow fatty acids to send all types of signals across the body. In contrast to saturated fatty acids, MUFAs and PUFAs are liquid at room temperature.

a) Monounsaturated Fatty Acids (MUFAs)

MUFAs are *not* essential fats; your body can produce them from the saturated fats already present in your body through a process called *de novo lipogenesis*. A key MUFA for overall health and athletic performance is called *oleic acid* (OA), composed of an 18-carbon chain with a double bond between carbons 9 and 10 (18:1w9). You can see the chemical structure of Oleic Acid in Figure 2.4.

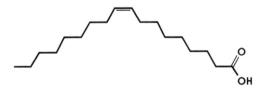

Figure 2.4. Chemical Structure of Oleic Acid

OA is the fat responsible for many of the beneficial properties of olive oil and avocados. It is also found in macadamia nuts, pistachios, pecans, peanuts, grape seed oil and almonds. OA plays a major role in keeping your arteries strong and supple, as well as being the predominant oil produced by skin glands.

Not all MUFAs are good for you. *Palmitoleic acid* (16:1w7) is a pro-inflammatory MUFA made in the body that is associated with increased risk of metabolic syndrome.[3] *Metabolic syndrome* is a medical condition diagnosed when a person displays three out of five of the following symptoms: high blood pressure, high triglycerides, high blood sugars, high abdominal fat or low HDL (good) cholesterol. Metabolic syndrome is alarmingly on the rise and a clear sign that your health is headed in the wrong direction.

TRANS-FATS, INFLAMMATION AND DISEASE

If your diet is high in processed sugars or processed foods, you are consuming an excess of trans fatty acids, which wreak havoc on the body. Trans-fats are made via a process called hydrogenation (the addition of a hydrogen atom) when processed food companies turn liquid fats into solid fats to extend the shelf life of processed foods and sugary treats.

Trans-fats can be found in a variety of foods such as margarine, crackers, cereal, candy, granola bars, salad dressing and fried food. Even what appear to be healthy foods such as wholegrain crackers or cereals can contain these bad fats. Research shows that the consumption of trans-fat laden donuts, French fries, fried chicken and candy are linked to increased inflammation and heart disease.[4]

In addition, when unsaturated fats are fried at high temperatures, the double bonds twist and form an unnatural and toxic trans-fat. For this reason, you should primarily use saturated fats like butter, ghee and coconut oil (no double bonds) for cooking. A Paleo diet is free of disease-causing trans-fats.

b) Polyunsaturated Fats (PUFAs)

While MUFAs are very important for athletes and overall health, polyunsaturated fatty acids play an even more significant role because they fulfil essential functions in the body. PUFAs are made up of two groups: omega-3 fats and omega-6 fats. Just like essential amino acids, obtaining optimal amounts of essential fatty acids (EFAs) omega-3 and omega-6 is critical for better health and productivity at work and in the gym, as well as achieving your weight loss and performance goals.

EFAs are critical for brain function and make up 30% of the one hundred billion brain cells (i.e., neurons) found in your brain. They also play a key role in building cell membranes and supporting immunity. EFAs strongly attract oxygen and play a vital role in the transfer of oxygen from the air to your lungs, from your lungs to your bloodstream, and ultimately from your red blood cells to hemoglobin—the oxygen carrier of the body. In this way, EFAs affect every cell in the body.

The Omega-6 Family

The omega-6 family of fatty acids is found in abundance in your average diet. The simplest omega-6 fat is called *linoleic acid* (LA, 18:2w6) and is made up of two double bonds (like a caterpillar bent in two places). See its chemical structure in Figure 2.5. LA is found primarily in vegetable oils, including corn, safflower, sunflower, sesame and many more.

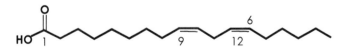

Figure 2.5. Chemical Structure of the Omega-6 Fat Linoleic Acid (LA, 18:2w6)

Another member of the omega-6 family includes *gamma-linoleic acid* (GLA, 18:3w). It's not normally present in most people's diets but found in borage, hemp and evening primrose oils. GLA reduces inflammation in the body via the production of hormone-like compounds called *prostaglandins*. Prostaglandins (PG) are short-lived compounds that regulate cellular activities on a moment-to-moment basis. They are made from essential fatty acids and exert a tremendous effect on the body. They are classified as series 1 (PGE1), series 2 (PGE2), and series 3 (PGE3). Series-1 prostaglandins are derived from the omega-6 fat *gamma-linoleic acid* (GLA) and carry out important functions in the body such as reducing inflammation, reducing joint pain, improving allergies and asthma, maintaining optimal immunity, supporting kidney function and keeping platelets from clotting.[5, 6, 7] PGE1 are considered the good prostaglandins.

Arachidonic acid (AA, 20:6w4) is a longer chain omega-6 fat found primarily in the fatty portion of meats. It was once thought that AA exerted mainly negative effects in the body, stimulating the production of series 2 prostaglandins (PG2) that play a key role in promoting inflammation. However, new research is revealing some beneficial effects of arachidonic acid and its role in reducing inflammation via conversion into a class of compounds called *lipoxins* and *resolvins*. Resolvins and lipoxins clean up the debris left over from the inflammatory reaction, which is critical for general health and performance.[8]

Arachidonic acid deficiency can result in hair loss, poor skin, mental disorders, and infertility. Like most things in life, it's all about the dose. The right amount of AA supports superior overall wellness and performance.

Omega-3 Family

In today's standard diet, omega-3 fats are much more difficult to obtain than omega-6 fats. The simplest omega-3 fatty acid is *alpha-linoleic acid* (ALA, 18:3w3), which has three double bonds and is commonly found in fish oil, seal oil, squid oil, sea algae and flaxseed oil. The body converts omega-3 fatty acids into longer and more highly unsaturated molecules, referred to as extra-long chain fatty acids like *eicosapentaneoic acid* (EPA, 20:5w3) and *decosahexanoic acid* (DHA, 22:6w3). In Figure 2.6, you can see how more double bonds lead to more kinks in the fatty acid chain.

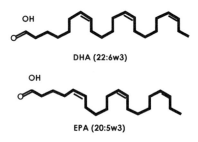

OH

DHA (22:6w3)

OH

EPA (20:5w3)

Figure 2.6. Chemical Structure of Decosahexanoic Acid (DHA,
22:6w3) and Eicosapentaneoic Acid (EPA, 20:5w3)

EPA and DHA are the omega-3 "all-stars" when it comes to improving overall health, recovery and athletic performance. They play essential roles in the body, cooling inflammatory pathways, improving brain and nervous system function, and supporting adrenal and sex gland hormone production.

While fish and seafood contain the richest sources of DHA and EPA, vegetarian sources of omega-3 fats include mechanically cold-pressed chia seeds, flax seeds, hemp seeds and walnut oils. However, a major drawback is that vegetarian sources do *not* convert very efficiently to EPA and DHA. Only fish oil, seal oil, krill oil and sea algae provide the necessary levels of DHA and EPA that you require to achieve your best health.

How important is DHA? It makes up about 90% of the omega-3 fats found in your brain and is the dominant fat found in breast milk (the healthiest food on earth!). It's also a key structural building block of cell membranes and plays a major role in controlling inflammation.

EPA exerts another important function in the body, stimulating the production of series 3 prostaglandins (PGE3). PGE3 share many of the positive health benefits of PGE1, but they also exert another important function—they *block* the production of "pro-inflammatory" PGE2s. This is a great example of how *both* an increase in omega-3 fats and a decrease in omega-6 are required to achieve optimal balance. A Paleo diet is naturally higher in omega-3 fats and lower in omega-6 fats, helping you achieve the desired ratio.

It's important to note that these beneficial prostaglandins require specific vitamins and minerals in order to be made from their EPA precursor. Adequate levels of vitamins C, B3, B6, and the minerals zinc and magnesium are necessary for the conversions to take place.

OMEGA-3 FATS AND MORTALITY

In 2013, the *Cardiovascular Healthy Study* examined over 2,500 individuals and showed that those people with the highest omega-3 (PUFA) levels in their blood had the lowest overall mortality rates.[9] The results showed the more omega-3 fats you eat, the less chance you have of dying from absolutely any cause! That sounds pretty convincing—pass the salmon, please!

OMEGA-3 FATS AND MUSCLE

A study at the *University of Washington* (2011) examined the effects of fish oil supplementation on muscle protein synthesis and key genetic signalling pathways associated with increasing lean muscle mass. Researchers found that fish oil supplementation resulted in an amazing 50% increase in the up-regulation of the mTOR genetic signalling pathways that control muscle growth.[10] Study participants had significant increases in muscle protein synthesis and muscular hypertrophy. (Evidence that healthy fats can make you strong, too!)

FAT DIGESTION

In contrast to proteins, the digestion of fats first takes place in the mouth as the enzyme *lingual lipase* initiates the breakdown of fats as you chew your food. Next, fats are further mixed in your stomach before travelling to your small intestine (duodenum) where bile is released from your gallbladder to emulsify the fats into smaller fat droplets.

At the same time, the enzyme *pancreatic lipase* is released from your pancreas to join in and help further break down fats. As the smaller fat droplets travel down to the final segment of your small intestine (ileum), they are packaged into compact bundles called *chylomicrons*, the water taxi carriers for fats. This process occurs so the fats can travel in the water-soluble environment (remember that fats in their initial form hate water) of your lymphatic system (immune system) to the capillaries (tiny blood vessels) before entering your liver. It is via the capillaries that fats enter into the cells of the body to produce energy, shown in Figure 2.7 below.

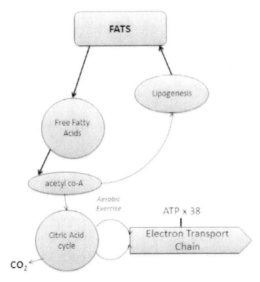

Figure 2.7 The Formation and Breakdown of Fats[11]

II. THE BIG DEBATE—THE <u>BEST</u> SOURCES OF FATS?

Coconut Oil

Coconut oil has been consumed for centuries as an integral part of a tropical diet and the coconut is so revered it's referred to as the "tree of life." It consists of 91% saturated fats and high levels of MCTs that are critical for optimal immune and digestive function. Coconut oil contains significant concentrations of lauric acid, a compound that exerts powerful antimicrobial effects. It also supports optimal testosterone levels, assists in the conversion of omega-3 fats into DHA, improves your blood lipid profile and protects the liver.

In Brazil, a recent study showed that people regularly consuming coconut oil had significantly less abdominal fat compared to placebo.[12] That's right! Coconut oil can help shrink your waistline. Another long-term clinical trial supports these findings, demonstrating the addition of MCT to the diet via coconut oil resulted in consistently less body fat accumulation.[13] Try adding one to two tablespoons to your morning breakfast shake, yogurt and oats or as a dip with fruit!

Red Palm Oil

Red palm oil is extracted from the fruit of the oil palm tree and is a nutritional powerhouse. It is packed with healthy short- and medium-chain saturated fats and its natural dark red colour makes it rich in beta-carotene and lycopene. Amazingly, raw red palm oil has 300 times more carotenoids than tomatoes!

Red palm oil is a great source of antioxidants, containing abundant concentrations of vitamin E and its more potent relatives the tocotrienols. However, stay away from the processed palm oil found in snack foods and baked goods because it acts like a trans-fatty acid and loses its health properties as well as its characteristic red colour.

Red palm oil is heat stable, like all saturated fats, so is safe to cook with at high temperatures. You can also add it on top of veggies and in your morning shake for a healthy antioxidant and energy boost!

Grass-fed Butter and Ghee

Butter is another healthy source of saturated fats that has a slightly different lipid profile compared to coconut oil, containing roughly 66% saturated fat and 33% monounsaturated fats. Butter is rich in butyric acid, the short-chain saturated fat with potent anti-microbial effects that supports superior immunity.

Another fat found abundantly in butter is a *trans-fat* but fear not, this one is good for you! Conjugated linoleic acid (CLA) is abundantly found in butter and the milk of *grass-fed* cows—about three to five times greater than traditional grain-fed cattle—helping to promote optimal health and stimulating weight loss.[14] Using full-fat cream is a great natural source of CLA.

Not everyone can digest butter. Although it contains virtually no lactose sugar, you may still have an allergic reaction to butter. This is due to the presence of the casein protein found in milk and butter. To remedy the situation, simply switch over to *clarified butter* or *ghee*. Ghee has been a staple of Indian cuisine for centuries and has all the same beneficial properties of butter without the casein!

Finally, butter from grass-fed cows contains high levels of vitamin K2, which supports better cardiovascular and bone health. How is K2 produced? The intestinal tracts of grass-fed cows ferment the vitamin K1 found in the leafy greens and grasses they graze on and convert it into the health-promoting vitamin K2. This is a major reason why healthy saturated fats are in fact beneficial for your heart.

Use butter or ghee to stir-fry or add it on to your veggies to get your daily dose of health-promoting short-chain fats.

Extra-virgin Olive Oil

Olive oil is rich in monounsaturated fats that contain the following:

- **Triterpenic acids**, which improve healing and exert anti-inflammatory effects

- **Caffeic** and **gallic acids,** which stimulate bile flow and improve elimination of toxins

- **Beta-sitosterol,** which lowers high cholesterol levels

- **Phenolic compounds**, which prevent the peroxidation (turning into toxic form) of fatty acids.[1]

It is important to consume the *extra-virgin* form of olive oil because this form is derived from the highest quality olives that are not damaged or bruised, and therefore contains no additional toxic chemical preservatives.

Other beneficial oil sources of MUFAs include macadamia oil, which contains a greater quantity of MUFAs than olive oil and is a good option for cooking (it can withstand temperatures up to 410°F). Try mixing these oils into your salad dressings, drizzling on top of veggies, or put a little into your morning shake to increase your healthy fat intake.

Avocados

Avocados are another great source of healthy monounsaturated fats. They also have major cholesterol-lowering effects on the body, decreasing your bad LDL cholesterol and increasing good HDL cholesterol. This is due to the presence of *beta-sitosterols*, a cholesterol-lowering nutrient that is now artificially added to processed foods to make them "healthier" (why not just get it from its natural source?).

Avocados are a terrific source of fibre and rich in vitamin A, folate, beta-carotene and the antioxidant lutein. Best of all, they have no effect on blood sugar levels! Try adding them to egg dishes at breakfast, with salads or meat servings at lunch or dinner, or in protein shakes to increase the healthy fat content.

Nuts

Walnuts have the most omega-3 fats of all nuts and contain significant amounts of *arginine*, a conditionally essential amino acid needed in greater concentrations during times of high stress or intense training. Arginine stimulates the production of nitric oxide, a compound that dilates blood vessels and improves blood flow to working muscles.

Macadamia nuts are another great choice for a snack during the day, as they also have one of the best ratios of omega-3 to omega-6. Originating in Australia and imported to Hawaii in the 1920s, they are a rich source of protein and fibre as well as chock full of electrolytes, potassium and calcium. Use walnuts and macadamia nuts as your snack of choice during the day.

Hemp Oil

Unrefined hemp oil ranges from dark to light green. It contains a beneficial ratio of healthy fats, 57% linoleic acid (omega-6) and 19% linolenic acid (omega-3 fats) in a more optimal ratio of 3:1. It also contains a considerable amount of the anti-inflammatory omega-6 fat GLA.

However, like all PUFAs make sure you do *not* cook with hemp oil. Simply mix it into your salad dressings, on top of your veggies, or into your protein shakes because it is a rich source of vitamins (B1, B3, B6) and minerals (calcium, magnesium, potassium).

Flax Oil

Flax oil is a golden colour and has a rich nutty taste. It is the richest source of omega-3 *alpha-linoleic acid* (ALA - 18:3w3); however, as I've mentioned before, it converts very poorly to extra-long chain fatty acids EPA and DHA, which are responsible for exerting many of the powerful health benefits of omega-3 fats on the body. Recent studies show that men convert only 8% and 4% of ALA into EPA and DHA respectively, while females fare a little better at 21% and 9%, respectively[15, 16]

Flax oil can be used to make salad dressings, added into protein shakes or drizzled on top of meals to support omega-3 intake. Do *not* fry or heat this oil; it spoils very easily when exposed to light, heat or oxygen.

Fish and Seafood Oils

Dietary sources of health promoting EPA and DHA are found abundantly in deep-sea, cold-water fatty fish such as black cod, salmon, mackerel, anchovies, sardines and herring. They are also found in crustaceans such as krill that are lower down on the food chain and therefore have less likelihood of heavy metal contamination.

You should consume a reasonable amount of fish and seafood from wild ocean sources to optimize your EPA and DHA intake. The extra-long-chain fatty acids provide many health benefits: reducing inflammation, stimulating lean muscle growth, supporting healthy heart function and promoting better mood and mental function. One serving of fish contains approximately 750–1,000mg of EPA, so be sure to include *at least* three servings per week.

MAMMALIAN OMEGA-3 FATS—SEAL OIL

The omega-3 fats found in fish, seafood and algae are slightly different from omega-3 fats found in mammals such as seals. Omega-3 fats from mammals can be absorbed directly in your mouth, due to the positioning of the free fatty acids on the glycerol backbone, thereby enhancing their bioavailability.[17, 18]

This is one of the major benefits of breast milk, allowing infants to absorb brain-building omega-3 fats directly in their mouths. New studies show this may be highly beneficial for people suffering from mood disorders or depression. How can you get mammalian omega-3 fats? Your best bet is to supplement with 1-2 capsules of seal oil daily.

Sea Algae

Sea algae are an excellent source of DHA omega-3 fatty acids. (Where do you think the fish get their daily dose of DHA?) Sea algae are lowest on the food chain, making it one of the purest sources of DHA and an excellent option for vegans and vegetarians. The only major drawback is that the supplemental form of sea algae DHA is not very potent, making it more expensive to achieve a therapeutic dose.

For vegetarians or vegans, be sure to include plenty of sea algae in your diet, as well as an algae source DHA supplement. It's important to note that DHA retro-converts very well to EPA (however EPA does not convert efficiently to DHA), so it should be your first choice for extra-long-chain omega-3 fats.

III. HOW THINGS GO WRONG

1) Too Many Omega-6 Fats

Omega-6 fats are typically found in over-abundance in the average person's diet. How is this possible? You unknowingly get too many omega-6 fats from processed foods, eating out at restaurants (most restaurants use omega-6 rich vegetable oils) and snack foods that are so readily available.

In today's standard diet, omega-3 fats (in particular EPA and DHA) are much more difficult to obtain in optimal amounts. The typical Western diet contains a ratio of omega-6 to omega-3 fats in the neighbourhood of 14:1-20:1, whereas research shows our Paleolithic ancestors had a much more balanced ratio in the neighbourhood of 2:1 to 1:1.[19] This imbalance is thought to be a major contributor to chronic inflammation and many of today's chronic degenerative diseases.[20,21] For athletes, this impairs your ability to recover from training or injury.

It's important to remember that you cannot just increase your DHA and EPA intake to correct your omega-3 to omega-6 imbalance. It's not that simple; more is not always better. You must also reduce your omega-6 intake. Ramping up omega-3 intake without reducing your omega-6s will not correct the imbalance due to a rate-limiting enzyme conversion in your body. Like most things in life, balance is the key.

TOO MANY OF THE WRONG NUTS

The nuts with the best ratio of omega-6 to omega-3 fats are walnuts and macadamia nuts, with ratios of 4:1 and 6:1 respectively. The next best on the list are pecans (21:1), pine nuts (32:1), cashews (48:1), and pistachios (52:1).[22] From here the ratios plummet rather quickly with Brazil nuts bringing up the rear at 378:1. Also, did you know that almonds have zero omega-3 fats!

If you are a nut-lover, try substituting walnuts, macadamia, pecans, pine nuts, and cashews for your regular snacks. You can still enjoy almonds a couple of times per week, but reducing your omega-6 intake will naturally restore a healthy balance of PUFAs.

2) Too Much Corn Oil

Corn oil ranks right up there with *trans-fats* on the *"fats to avoid"* list. Omega-6 rich corn oil is pro-inflammatory due to its lipid peroxidation, a process where free radicals steal electrons from your cell membranes, leading to cellular damage. Peroxidation affects polyunsaturated fats much more strongly than saturated fats because they have more double bonds. Reducing your omega-6 intake reduces your overall peroxidation levels.

You might be thinking, "I never eat corn oil," but the reality is you probably do; you just don't realize it. For example, corn oil is used in most restaurants to fry vegetables and meats because of its high smoking point. If you've ever eaten French fries, chances are they were deep-fried in corn oil (studies shows over 70% of fast food chains use pro-inflammatory corn oil). If you want to reduce your corn oil and omega-6 intake, switch over to a wholefood-based diet, avoid deep-fried foods and limit the amount of processed foods that come in wrappers, packages or boxes. In other words, adopt a more Paleo dietary approach!

3) Not Enough Saturated Fats

Saturated fats play a key role in supporting better overall health and performance. They help mitigate reductions in testosterone levels that stem from busy work schedules, mental stress or intense training. Athletes consuming insufficient saturated fats suffer from significant decreases in testosterone levels after intense training.[23] In clinical practice, almost three-quarters of patients test positive for low levels of free testosterone.

Testosterone is your powerful muscle building, fat-burning and mood-enhancing hormone. It is as important for women as it is for men. If your testosterone levels are running on empty, your health, weight loss and performance goals will suffer (along with your libido!).

MCTs found in saturated fats such as coconut oil also assist in liver detoxification pathways (Phase I/II) that help to expel toxins from the body and keep your liver cells healthy. If you are consuming alcohol, coffee, prescription drugs or fast foods on a regular basis, your liver will be working overtime.

Finally, MCTs are the primary fuel for your enterocytes or gut cells, helping to keep your digestive system strong. The powerful antimicrobial effects of healthy saturated fats found in coconut oil, grass-fed butter and ghee help to support the ideal environment for good gut bacteria to thrive in the gut.

4) You Are Scared of Animal Fat

Animal fats have gotten a bad rap over the last few decades because many doctors and health experts have continued to hammer home the message that they will clog your arteries and lead to cardiovascular disease. Is this really the case? Should animal fats really be avoided like the plague?

Animal fats are loaded with fat-soluble vitamins A, D, E and K—all of which are extremely important for immunity, cardiovascular health and overall wellness. The interesting thing is that many of these fat-soluble vitamins are not easy to obtain from most foods, a major reason why deficiencies of these vitamins are so commonplace.

The best sources of fat-soluble vitamins are seafood, dairy, organ meats, eggs and insects (don't worry, you can stick with the first four!). Animal fat is high in choline, a precursor to the neurotransmitter acetylcholine, which is essential for optimal brain health.

Another common mistake is *not* eating your egg yolks. The fear of artery clogging fat, high cholesterol levels and too many calories has led people to believe they should be avoided. Nothing could be further from the truth. The egg yolk is arguably the most nutritious part of the egg! One yolk provides you with 245 IUs of immune-boosting vitamin A and is one of the few food sources of vitamin D! As well, the yolk is loaded with choline that supports better brain function and protects you against heart disease.

If you want better health and performance, eat the whole egg and healthy animal fats, staples of a Modern Paleo diet. It's not the eggs that cause health problems, it's all the carbs (toast, pancakes, muffins, cereals, fruit juice) served along with it that should be limited if you are overweight or struggling with your health.

IV. THE BENEFITS OF A HIGH FAT DIET (AKA MODERN PALEO DIET)

The benefits of a high fat diet are extremely diverse and well documented in the scientific literature. Achieving your optimal intake of healthy fats helps cool inflammation, improve endurance, blunt cortisol stress levels, shed body fat, balance hormones and improve joint pain.

Fats and Muscular Recovery

A study at the *University of Florida* recruited 40 untrained males, between the ages of 18 and 35, who performed rigorous training regimes over a two-week period. Half of the trainees received omega-3 DHA supplements with added vitamin E and flavonoids, while the other half received a placebo. The results showed that consuming DHA supplements after exercise *significantly reduced muscular inflammation* (lab markers IL-6 and CRP).[24] Cooling inflammation post-training is important to prevent excessive muscular damage and accelerate recovery between workouts.

Fats and Exercise Endurance

In Japan, a study investigated the effects of two weeks of MCT consumption on exercise endurance. The results showed that athletes consuming MCTs were able to *suppress elevations in lactic acid levels* compared to the placebo group.[25] They also experienced longer time to exhaustion, an important benefit for athletes and especially endurance athletes!

Fats and Mental Stress

In England, the *British Journal of Nutrition* discovered that supplementing with a combination of EPA + DHA (1.8g) helped *reduce the adrenal over-activation* associated with high levels of mental stress.[26] This type of adrenal over-activation or stress is even more common now in the workplace with constant connectivity and access via mobile Internet devices.

In Germany, a recent study demonstrated that supplementing with omega-3 fats plus *phosphatidylserine* (PS)—a phospholipid found on the inner membrane of cells—lowered the indices of chronic and acute stress by supporting the hypothalamus-pituitary-adrenal (HPA) axis.[27] The HPA axis is a complex set of feedback mechanisms between your brain and your adrenal glands that control your body's reaction to stress (more on this in Chapter 8—Cortisol). Limiting excessive or prolonged cortisol output is extremely important for accelerating recovery, whether from exercise or the constant stress of work.

Fats and Weight Loss

In France, researchers examined the effect of fish oil supplementation on blood sugar and insulin levels. Researchers found EPA + DHA (1.8g) fish oil supplementation over a three-week period resulted in *significant improvements in insulin function.*[28] This is extremely important for long-term weight loss; high insulin levels are associated with weight gain, excess body-fat accumulation and poor health.

Fats and Sex Hormones

The *National Cancer Institute* in Maryland conducted a study of 43 men and measured the effects of healthy dietary fats and fibre consumption on circulating levels of the sex hormones testosterone and estrogen. After a 10-week period, people eating the high-fat and high-fibre diet showed *dramatic increases in testosterone* production (13%), while simultaneously reducing estrogen levels (12-28%).[29] This clearly shows the tremendous effect fats can have on hormonal balance.

Fats and Joint Pain

In Wales, researchers at *Cardiff University* found that supplemental EPA and DHA were able to reduce key proteins that trigger the disease progression in osteoarthritis.[30] There is an important relationship between omega-3 fats, genetic messenger RNA (responsible for converting your DNA into specific amino acids) and their impact on osteoarthritis.

EPA provides anti-inflammatory support by *blocking* pro-inflammatory PGE2s, reducing pro-inflammatory markers *interleukin-6* (IL-6) and *tumour-necrosis factor* alpha (TNF-a), and increasing production of *resolvins* and *protectins.*[31] All of these compounds help to reduce inflammation and clear out the cellular debris caused by inflammation—important for anyone suffering from pain.

Fats and Depression

Athletes are not immune to mood affective disorders. In fact, one of the principal signs of overtraining is irritability and depressed mood. Recent studies from leading European medical journals show that people experiencing depression have consistently lower levels of essential fatty acids in their blood. Supplementation with fish oils resulted in a significant improvement in the Hamilton Rating Scale for Depression, a recognized evaluation system for depression.[32] EPA has been shown in multiple trials to support positive outcomes from mood disorders and depression.[33]

Those people experiencing mood and depressive episodes should have their omega-3 levels assessed (along with vitamin D) in order to correct possible nutritional deficiencies that may be causing or exacerbating their condition.

V. THE PALEO PROJECT—FAT SOLUTIONS

You should aim to consume optimal amounts of *healthy* fats to support your goals to look, feel and perform your best. Check out Figure 2.8 for a list of healthy fats to consider. Typically, the ratio should consist of one-third saturated fats, one-third MUFAs and one-third PUFAs. Your intake should be derived from a variety of food sources in order to meet your daily requirements.

SATURATED FATS	MUFAS	PUFAS
Coconut oil Red palm oil Butter Ghee (clarified butter)	Olive oil (Extra-Virgin) Avocado Macadamia nut oil	Fish oils Mammalian oils Sea algae Flax oil Walnut oil Hemp oil
* These are very heat stable oils, excellent for cooking at high temperatures	* These are somewhat heat stable oils, safe for low-heat cooking	* Do NOT cook with these oils. Use in salad dressings or on top of veggies

Figure 2.8. Summary of Healthy Fats

Check out Figure 2.9 for your *Fat Solutions Action Plan*. Review the list of objectives and incorporate all the action plan points to continue building your Modern Paleo diet, the nutritional foundation for better health, a better body and better performance.

FAT SOLUTIONS ACTION PLAN

1. Consume 1-3 tbsp PUFAs daily
- Divided equally between meals throughout the day. Includes fish, krill, sea algae, walnut, hemp, flax and mammalian oils. Do not cook with these.

2. Consume 1-3 tbsp MUFAs daily
- Divided equally between meals throughout the day. Includes extra-virgin olive oil, macadamia nut oil and avocado. Safe for low-heat cooking.

3. Consume 1-3 tbsp of healthy saturated fats daily
- Divided equally between meals throughout the day. Includes coconut oil, butter, ghee and red palm oil. All excellent for cooking at high temps.

4. Reduce your intake of omega-6 fats
- Limit processed foods and excessive intake of vegetable oils.

Figure 2.9. Healthy Fats Action Plan

SAMPLE MENU

Listed below are various options for increasing your healthy fats intake through the day. You can cook with the fats or simply add them on top of your dishes. One serving of fats is roughly equivalent to one thumb-size portion of fat (or 1 tbsp). Women should aim for one thumb per meal, while men should aim for two. As you move to the next chapter, I'll round out your diet with suggestions for carbohydrate intake.

Breakfast Options

1. Eggs (4-6 for men; 2-4 for women) + avocado

2. Protein shake (30-40g) + coconut oil

3. Chicken breast (or any other meat) + grass-fed butter

4. Vegetarian option – Full-fat plain yogurt (1 cup)

Snacks (AM)

- Walnuts (approximately 7-8 nuts)

- Full-fat yogurt (approximately 1 cup)

Lunch Options

1. Salmon fillet + avocado

2. Grass-fed beef + macadamia oil

3. Turkey breast + olive oil

4. Vegetarian option – tempeh + coconut oil

Snacks (PM)

- Macadamia nuts (approximately 7-8 nuts)

- Kefir (approximately 1 cup)

Dinner Options

1. Pork + red palm oil

2. Black cod + olive oil

3. Bison + ghee

4. Vegetarian option – yellow lentils + ghee

CHAPTER 3

CARBOHYDRATES—The Athlete's Fuel

You don't need to look any further than the breakfast table to see how prevalent carbs are in our diets. Most people start their day with some combination of orange juice, cereal, toast, muesli, granola or bagel. While this might be a healthy option for some, for most people it will lead them down the path to weight gain, poor performance and worsening health.

The typical Western diet is loaded with processed and simple carbohydrates that can quickly send your blood sugars on a rollercoaster ride through the day. Unfortunately, these peaks and valleys accelerate weight gain and sabotage your health.

A diet high in sugars and carbs exacerbates most chronic diseases such as diabetes, high blood pressure, high cholesterol, heart disease and many cancers. This has led to a new movement in recent years toward lower carb diets, with a new belief that a low-carb approach is healthiest for everyone.

However, your optimal carbohydrate consumption is more complex than this. It depends on your current level of activity, general health, genetics and personal goals (weight loss, performance or better overall health). These factors must be taken into account in order to develop a personalized diet that's right for you.

The *amount* and *type* of carbohydrates you choose to eat—as well as *when* you choose to eat them—play a strong role in determining your body composition, building lean muscle and supporting better health. Your total carb intake will vary markedly if you are training for performance versus if you are trying to get leaner.

In this chapter, I will outline how to choose the best sources of carbohydrates to support your goals and show common pitfalls that sabotage your health, weight-loss progress or performance in the gym.

I. BACK TO BASICS—CARBOHYDRATES 101

The scientific term for carbohydrates is *saccharides*. They can be divided into three general groups: monosaccharides, disaccharides, and polysaccharides. Monosaccharides are the simplest form of carbohydrate consisting of only one sugar and generally have a sweet taste. You probably eat some monosaccharides every day in the form of *glucose* (starches), *fructose* (fruit) and *galactose* (milk). Figure 3.1 shows you the chemical structure of all three monosaccharides.

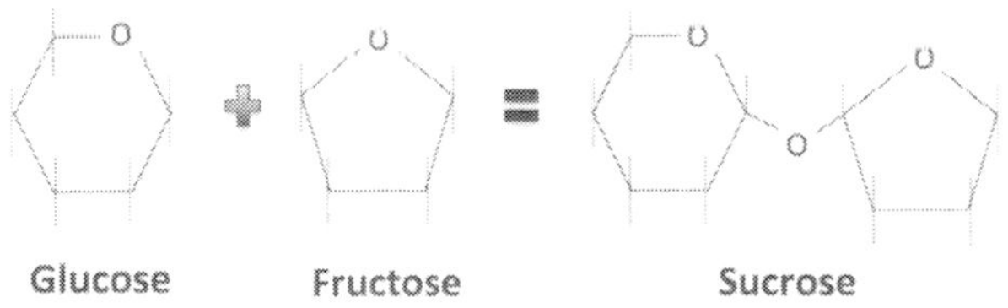

Glucose   Fructose   Sucrose

Figure 3.1. Chemical Structure of Glucose, Fructose and Sucrose

Monosaccharides

The main energy currency of your body is *glucose*, which is rapidly absorbed into your bloodstream. It is found naturally in your diet from more complex starches such as rice, grains, pastas, potatoes and root vegetables that contain multiple glucose molecules linked together.

After you've eaten a serving of carbs, glucose in the body has three possible fates:

- Used as fuel for activity or exercise

- Stored as glycogen, the carb reserves in your muscles and liver

- Converted to body fat

Three simple fates—burn it, add it to muscle or store it as fat. That's it.

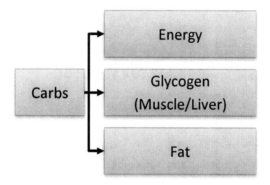

Figure 3.2. Three Possible Fates of Carbohydrates (Glucose)

You can think of complex carbohydrates as the fuel you put in your car's gas tank. The more you drive, the more fuel you need. The less you drive, the less fuel you need. The x-factor is the *type of carbs* you are consuming because they can have very different effects on your body (more on this later in the chapter).

Fructose is another common monosaccharide that you probably eat every day. It's found primarily in fruit, natural sweeteners such as honey and processed sweeteners such as high-fructose corn syrup (HFCS). Like glucose, fructose is a quick fuel source for the body.

However, fructose is not your body's preferred energy source. It must be *converted* into glucose in your liver before you can use it as a fuel for activity. This reaction takes time, making fructose less desirable than glucose for instant energy during exercise. Also, fructose is preferentially stored in your liver (as liver glycogen), while glucose is stored in your muscle tissue (as muscle glycogen). You have approximately four times the capacity to store muscle glycogen compared to liver glycogen. You see later in this chapter how saturating liver glycogen can dramatically affect weight gain.

Disaccharides

Disaccharide sugars are made up of two monosaccharide sugars linked together. They are naturally found in cane sugar, fruit, vegetables or table sugar. *Sucrose* is a disaccharide formed when one fructose molecule is linked to one glucose molecule (see figure 3.1). It's the sugar most commonly used in popular sports drinks to provide energy to working muscles.

Lactose is a disaccharide naturally found in milk that helps babies grow into children and young adults. However, people tend to lose the ability to digest this sugar when they reach adulthood. This is why *lactose intolerance* or the inability to digest lactose is so commonplace and can lead to gas, bloating and digestive discomfort. Finally, *maltose* is another disaccharide commonly found in cereals, pastas, potatoes and beer!

Polysaccharides

Polysaccharides are complex carbohydrate molecules, containing more than ten monosaccharide units linked together, like branches of a tree. Complex carbs are broken down slowly and steadily into glucose subunits to fuel activity or exercise and can be stored as glycogen. Examples of polysaccharide-rich foods include starchy root vegetables and tubers (vegetables that grow below ground), rice, potatoes, grains and corn. All of these are traditional staples in diets across the globe.

Another important type of polysaccharide for good health is *cellulose*. Cellulose is not an energy source for the body but an *indigestible fibre* that forms the basic cellular structure of vegetables and fruit. Although it does not directly provide the body with nutrients, cellulose's high fibre content helps to *slow the release of carbohydrates* during meals, keeps the bowel moving properly and promotes the growth of healthy intestinal microflora (which produce essential vitamins).

Finally, polysaccharides include *soluble fibre* such as *pectins* commonly found in apples, oranges, nuts and oats. Soluble fibres form a gel-like substance that delays gastric emptying, putting the brakes on the release of glucose into your blood stream and thereby supporting a slow and steady release of energy and increased satiety. All of these are key factors in supporting weight loss, better performance and better health.

Carbohydrate Digestion
Whereas protein digestion primarily takes place in the stomach, carbohydrate digestion starts as soon as food enters your mouth. Your first bite kick-starts the production of *salivary amylase*, the enzyme that initiates the breakdown of complex starches into simpler disaccharides. This is a key reason why chewing your food thoroughly is so important!

As your food moves down into the stomach, it's further churned and mixed before moving into your small intestine, where your pancreas releases the enzyme *pancreatic amylase* to help further breakdown the starches. The majority of your carbohydrate digestion takes place in your mouth and small intestine, so if you don't digest them properly, it can wreak havoc on your gut and the balance of good and bad gut bacteria (more on this in Chapter 4—Digestion).

All along the surface of your small intestine there are tiny projections called *intestinal microvilli*, which increase the surface area of your gut to maximize absorption. These microvilli contain vital digestive enzymes—*lactase*, *maltase* and *sucrose*—that deliver the final blow and break down disaccharides into their most easily absorbable monosaccharide form. The microvilli then soak up the fully digested simple carbs into your bloodstream.

Carbohydrates and the Glycemic Index
The glycemic index (GI), shown in Figure 3.3, is a ranking system that reflects how quickly foods (proteins, fats and carbohydrates) are taken

up into your bloodstream. Carbohydrates have *the greatest impact on the glycemic index*; therefore, knowing which carbs are quickly absorbed (high GI) versus those that are more slowly absorbed (low GI) is crucial in optimizing your performance in the gym, accelerating fat loss and improving your overall health.

For example, high-glycemic carbs such as white potatoes or bagels are rapidly absorbed into your bloodstream, spiking blood sugar levels as well as your blood sugar hormone insulin. In contrast, low glycemic carbs such as apples or oats enter the bloodstream slowly and steadily over a longer period of time.

Low-Glycemic Foods (0-50)	Mid-Glycemic Foods (50-70)	High-Glycemic Foods (70+)
Meats – 0	Sweet potato – 54	Bagel – 72
Fats – 0	Brown Rice – 55	Mashed potatoes – 73
Vegetables (non-starch) < 15	Yucca – 55	Cheerios cereal – 74
Whole Milk – 27	Plantains – 55	White bread – 79
Chocolate Milk – 34	Kidney beans – 56	Rice cakes – 82
Apple – 36	Table sugar – 65	Cornflakes – 84
Whole Wheat Spaghetti – 36	Rye bread – 65	*Baked* Sweet potato – 94
Chickpeas – 42	*Instant* Oats – 66	Parsnips – 98
Whole Oats – 50	Whole wheat bread – 68	Dates – 100

Figure 3.3. GI Index Table

Incorporating foods rich in soluble fibre is important in slowing down the release of sugars into your bloodstream, as well as maintaining healthy gut function. The average North American gets about 5g of fibre in his diet daily—a long way off the recommended 25g per day by the National Cancer Institute and even further away from the estimated 40-50g that Paleolithic ancestors regularly consumed in their primitive diets.[2] Excellent sources of soluble fibre include oats, Brussels sprouts, sweet potatoes, turnips, asparagus and ground flaxseeds.

In general, foods higher in protein, fibre (i.e., veggies and fruit) and healthy fats tend to have a lower glycemic index and should be the focal point of a healthy diet. A Modern Paleo diet optimizes your intake of all these foods. High-glycemic foods should be prioritized during or after exercise. Learning *when* to consume specific carbs, referred to as *nutrient timing,* is critical for supporting superior weight loss and performance (more on this in Section III—Performance).

WHAT'S WRONG WITH ORANGE JUICE FOR BREAKFAST?

Orange juice is a classic staple in a North American breakfast. Unfortunately, about 75% of the population (those overweight and obese) should NOT be consuming juice for breakfast or at any time of the day! Orange juice is rapidly absorbed into your bloodstream, leading to spikes in blood sugar and insulin levels. If you are overweight, your insulin function is unlikely to be up to par and high-GI drinks like orange juice can worsen blood sugar levels and result in unwanted weight gain and worsening health.

Carbohydrates and Insulin

The hormone insulin is your primary blood sugar hormone. It's produced in your pancreas and its main role is to get carbohydrates from your bloodstream into your cells. It accomplishes this task by signalling your cells to absorb glucose via specific receptors called *glucose transporters* (GLUT). There are various types of GLUT receptors; some are located on the cell surface and are always ready to absorb glucose.

GLUT-3 receptors are located in your brain and because your brain needs a steady stream of glucose for you to survive, these receptors are constantly able to absorb glucose. In contrast, GLUT-4 receptors are located *inside* your cells and need to be coaxed up to your cells' surface to absorb glucose. Exercise and activity stimulates the GLUT4 receptors to come up to the cell surface during and after exercise to preferentially soak up the carbs!

Insulin is also a powerful anabolic hormone; it helps to *build*. It can help you build lean muscle or it can help you build fat! It's all about timing. If you are exercising regularly, you can harness the power of insulin to help build lean muscle and recover more quickly from training. However, if you are out of shape or overweight, chronically elevated insulin levels will promote weight gain and increased body fat. It all depends on the individual.

Carbohydrates have the greatest impact on the glycemic index of foods and therefore have the greatest impact on insulin output. Insulin release is proportional to the speed of carbohydrate absorption into the bloodstream. As a result, quickly absorbed high-GI foods cause a rush of sugars into the blood and a subsequent surge of insulin. Low-GI foods are slowly and steadily absorbed into the bloodstream, leading to a gradual release of insulin.

II. THE BIG DEBATE—THE <u>BEST</u> SOURCES OF CARBOHYDRATES

The ideal sources of complex carbohydrates for athletes, active people and those striving for better health should come from "clean" or gluten-free carbs. Food allergies can lead to a whole host of problems that sabotage your health, weight loss and performance goals, so it's important to select carbohydrate sources that are *hypo-allergenic* (I go into more detail in Chapter 4—Digestion and Chapter 5—Immunity).

In clinical practice, clients see dramatic improvements in energy levels, recovery time, immunity and performance after shifting away from processed and allergenic foods. This trend has taken root with many elite athletes, most notably with respect to the elimination of wheat and gluten from their diets.

Clean carbs are found in abundance in a Paleo diet because our hunter-gatherer ancestors evolved eating gluten-free carbs—root vegetables, tubers and broadleaf plants—*before* the agricultural revolution and introduction of wheat and gluten 10,000 years ago. A Modern Paleo approach has a few exceptions to the original plan, based on what the latest science is telling us. The following sections list nutrient-dense, high-quality complex carbohydrate choices ideal for optimal health and performance. The best strategy is to include a variety of carbs to ensure a robust intake of essential vitamins and minerals.

ROOTS AND TUBERS

Roots and tuberous vegetables have been staple foods for people in Africa, Asia and Latin America for centuries. They provide a naturally gluten-free source of carbohydrate that is tremendously nutrient dense, loaded with vitamins, minerals and essential nutrients.

Sweet Potato

Sweet potatoes are a terrific carbohydrate source, providing a slow release of energy when boiled or a high-glycemic burst when baked. They are rich in fibre and the orange pigment is loaded with immune-boosting vitamin A, helping to keep colds and flu at bay. Sweet potato contains *vitamin-B6 (pyridoxine)* to support BCAA metabolism, potassium for electrolyte balance and powerful antioxidant vitamins C and E. The glycemic index of *boiled* sweet potatoes is 46, while *baked* sweet potatoes tip the GI scale at 94.

Yams

Often confused with sweet potatoes, yams come from the plant family *Dioscoreacea*, while sweet potatoes are from the *Convolvulaceae* family (make sure to wow your friends at the next cocktail party with that one!). Yams are a dietary staple on four continents and like most *roots and tubers* are highly nutritious. Yams have significant amounts of vitamins C and B6 and are exceptionally high in potassium, making them a great source of electrolytes after exercise. The glycemic index for yams is 54 and, like sweet potatoes, they can be baked to boost the glycemic index.

Yucca (Cassava)

Yucca is high in B-vitamins that are essential for converting proteins, carbs and fats into energy. One cup of yucca root packs a 42mg punch of vitamin C, crucial for collagen formation to keep your joints healthy and immune system strong. Yucca root contains *resveratrol*, a natural anti-inflammatory and anti-oxidant that protects your body from damage caused by free radicals (these are produced during exercise—like the exhaust that comes out of your car when you drive).

Fat-soluble antioxidant vitamins A and E are found in yucca and the glycemic index is 55.

Jicama

This white-fleshed tuber is a staple in Mexican and South American cuisine. It is relatively bland tasting and is commonly served with lime and chillies. Jicama is a low-calorie, low-glycemic, high-fibre root veggie loaded with calcium, vitamin C, magnesium, vitamin A and beta-carotene. You can boil or bake it and add it to virtually any dish.

Plantains

Plantains and bananas come from the same *Musa* plant family but are quite different. Plantains must be cooked and are a much denser source of carbohydrate. Plantains can be boiled, baked or fried and have been staples in African and Caribbean cultures for centuries. They are loaded with potassium—a whopping 720mg per cup—that is crucial for replenishing electrolytes after exercise. Plantains are a great source of vitamins A, B3, C and fibre (3.5g/cup).

Turnips, Parsnips, Rutabaga, Carrots and Beets

Other root vegetables such as turnips, parsnips, rutabaga, carrots and beets are all terrific sources of nutrient-dense complex carbohydrates. For example, turnips provide a robust 240mg of potassium, 3g of fibre and 20mg of vitamin C per cup. Parsnips provide a nice sweet taste to go along with generous amounts of folate, calcium, potassium and a group of phytochemicals called *phthalides,* which inhibit inflammatory enzymes.

Rutabagas are a cross between turnips and wild cabbage and pack a massive potassium punch with almost 800mg per cup, along with 4g of fibre and over 50mg of magnesium.

Beets are a root vegetable revered in Eastern medicine for their ability to cleanse the liver and purify the blood. Not surprisingly, beets are rich in dietary nitrates that have been shown to improve aerobic work capacity by as much as 20%! They are a terrific source of betaine and folate, which work together to keep your heart and blood vessels strong.

Finally, carrots are a classic root vegetable staple that are loaded with immune-boosting vitamin A (three carrots contain 30,000 IUs of vitamin A) as well as high concentrations of the antioxidant beta-carotene, which is associated with a decreased risk of many types of cancers.

Root vegetables add a colourful palette to your plate and are very versatile. Boil or steam them for a low to mid-GI effect or bake them for a high-GI meal after exercise.

PSEUDO-CEREALS

True cereal grains are grasses, whereas *pseudo-cereal grains* are broadleaf plants (non-grasses) that can be used in a similar way to traditional grains. The benefit is that they are typically much more nutrient dense and are much less likely to cause food allergy reactions. The pseudo-cereals are fantastic carb options in a Modern Paleo diet.

Quinoa

This ancient grain from the Inca trail is a nutritional powerhouse and has gained much attention over the past few years. Quinoa (pronounced *keen-wa*) contains all essential amino acids and has 50% more protein compared to wheat containing carbohydrates. It is prepared very easily and is great option for pre-workout meals. The glycemic index of quinoa is very low at 35.

Amaranth

An ancient grain originating from the Aztec populations, amaranth is renowned for its ability to strengthen the lungs, especially important for endurance athletes. It is also loaded with nutrients and is another gluten-free complex carbohydrate option. One cup provides 10g of protein (very high for a grain) and is actually higher in calcium and magnesium than cow's milk! It has a sticky texture and therefore makes a great option for a hot breakfast cereal. The glycemic index of amaranth is very low.

Buckwheat

This pseudo-cereal is a little confusing. Although it contains the word "wheat" in its name, buckwheat is a broadleaf plant and NOT a grass related to wheat. In Asia, buckwheat noodles have been a culinary staple for centuries in Japan, China and Korea. Buckwheat has a low-GI score. It contains more protein than rice, wheat or millet and is rich in magnesium, the flavonoid rutin and fibre. Buckwheat helps to improve your cholesterol profile, lowering your total and bad LDL cholesterol and increasing good HDL cholesterol.[3]

CEREAL GRAINS

Although technically not allowed in a classic Paleo diet, I support the use of certain cereal grains (depending on the individual and tolerance) in a Modern Paleo diet based on the benefits I've seen in clinical practice. This is a controversial topic in the Paleo world, with hardline Paleo followers avoiding them completely.

I believe a Modern Paleo approach integrates foods that are highly nutritious, gluten-free and hypo-allergenic (i.e., don't typically lead to adverse allergic reactions). If a food provides more benefits than drawbacks, does not sacrifice health and performance, and makes it easier for more people to join the Paleo movement then it should be included in your diet. The Modern Paleo approach is your platform from which to *personalize* the best diet for *you*.

Brown Rice

Highly beneficial for your digestive and nervous systems, this cereal grain is a terrific match for athletes because training places a heavy burden on these systems. Rice is a hypo-allergenic grain that is easily digested and rarely triggers food allergies. Traditional Chinese medicine (TCM) recommends consuming short-grain brown rice in the winter months to keep your system *warmed* and long-grain in the summer to *cool* your body. The glycemic index of brown rice is 55, compared to 72 for white rice, and 87 for instant rice.

Wild Rice

Native to the North American marsh grasses, this form of rice is higher in iron, B-vitamins and protein than brown rice. It's an excellent low glycemic carbohydrate that can be consumed before training to provide a slow and steady release of energy. The glycemic index of wild rice (57) is approximately the same as brown rice.

Oats

Oats are classified as *nervines* in herbal medicine texts, meaning they have a superb ability to support the nervous system. During intense exercise or busy days at work your nervous system is heavily taxed, making oats a wonderful tonic to help the body recover, especially during winter months. *Steel-cut oats* are the only truly *gluten-free* oat and contain double the amount of protein and fibre compared to regular oats. Whole oats (glycemic index of 51) are more slowly absorbed compared to quick oats, which are taken up more rapidly into the bloodstream (glycemic index of 66). **Note**: Regular oats do not naturally contain gluten but are typically made in the same facilities as gluten containing grains and therefore are not considered gluten-free.)

Millet

Millet is another excellent gluten-free grain option and a nutritious choice for meeting your total daily carbohydrate requirements on a gluten-free diet. Millet is very high in magnesium, potassium, B-vitamins and vitamin E. Millet supports the digestive system and provides a slow-sustained energy supply to the body with a glycemic index of 25.

VEGETABLES AND FRUIT

Many people don't realize that vegetables and fruit are classified as carbohydrates. Typically, I tell my clients to eat *unlimited* amounts of vegetables because they are tremendously nutrient dense and very low in calories. (Have you ever tried to eat a head of broccoli in one sitting? It's much more difficult than eating a bag of jellybeans!). This is a major benefit of adopting a Paleo diet—it forces you to eat more vegetables!

As for fruit, it really depends on the individual. If you are already lean and training regularly then your intake can be on the higher end. However if you are trying to lose weight and shed body fat, then reducing your fruit intake or eliminating it completely may be advised (more on this in Chapter 9—Upgrade Your Body).

SHOULD I INCLUDE BEANS IN MY DIET?

For athletes who want to increase their carbohydrate or caloric intake, beans are a beneficial source of complex carbohydrates that provide sustained-release energy due to their high fibre content. However, there are some major drawbacks from eating too many beans.

Beans contain a whole host of anti-nutrients, including lectins and phytates that negatively affect the body. In nature, plants are armed with anti-nutrients to ward off being eaten by foraging animals, but they can also irritate humans. For example, lectins are a substance known to damage the lining of the human gut and can induce dramatic shifts in bacterial flora, increase intestinal permeability and impair immune system function.[4] Phytates bind minerals and reduce your ability to absorb key nutrients such as magnesium, zinc, calcium and iron. Therefore, try to limit bean consumption in your diet (or eliminate them entirely). Substitute lentils or eat beans cooked to destroy most of the anti-nutrients.

III. HOW THINGS GO WRONG

1) Too Many Carbs (Especially White Carbs)

Compared to proteins and fat, carbohydrates have the most profound impact on weight gain. Eating too many carbs—especially white carbs, sweets and simple sugars—forces your body to pump out a surge of insulin to cope with the rapid rise in blood sugar. Eventually your pancreas can't keep up the insulin production and the result is poor insulin efficiency or *insulin resistance*. This is the point where many people get stuck in the weight-gain cycle.

Controlling carbohydrate intake is critical for your long-term health and weight loss. In general, the more overweight or unhealthy you are, the poorer your insulin sensitivity. This means your body will need to pump out greater concentrations of insulin to offset your poor insulin function. The overwhelming consensus among expert researchers is that the intake of excess carbohydrates is the driving force behind insulin dysfunction, weight gain and worsening health (more on this in Chapter 7—Insulin).

2) Too Much Fructose

Fructose is the sugar naturally found in fruit. When added to soda pop and desserts, it acts differently in the body. Too much fructose will make you fat. Experts now agree that the increasing prevalence of processed snack foods loaded with high-fructose corn syrup (HFCS) has led to the increasing weight gain and obesity levels in the general population.

A growing body of scientific evidence supports the notion that the excess intake of HFCS—via sweetened beverages and processed snacks—is associated with increased body weight and the increased incidence of metabolic and cardiovascular disorders.[11] If improved health and body composition is your goal, you must avoid fructose sweeteners found in snack foods, candy or processed foods.

Too much fructose in your diet disrupts the balance of good and bad intestinal microflora in your gut. In Switzerland, a recent study from the *Institute of Food* found a connection between high fructose intake, altered gut bacteria and subsequent gain in weight[12] (more on this in Chapter 4—Digestion).

HFCS is used in almost all processed foods or sweets and often labelled as a *natural sweetener*. Unfortunately, it is not natural to consume fructose in such great quantities! Therefore, if you want to improve body composition and upgrade your health you must *avoid* HFCS and limit fruit consumption if you are overweight (eliminate completely if obese).

3) Too Much Soda Pop

Are you a regular soda pop drinker? Do you drink a can of soda daily to help get you through the workday or give you some energy to exercise? If this sounds like you, you are putting your health in danger. Did you know that regular pop consumption increases your cardiovascular disease risk by a whopping 20%, according to the *Harvard School of Public Health!*[13] These sugary drinks affect your cholesterol levels, alter your satiety hormone leptin and cause inflammation.

Not surprisingly, the authors of the study go on to state that the high consumption of soda pop is associated with increased weight gain and metabolic diseases. They believe the only beverages you should be drinking are water, tea and coffee (in moderation). That's it—straight from the experts!

4) Too Much Alcohol

When I ask patients if they ever binge-drink, the answer is usually an emphatic "No." However, most people don't know the medical definition of binge drinking. Binge drinking is defined as consuming four or more drinks in one sitting for women and five or more drinks for men. Based on this definition, a recent study showed one in six people binge-drink four times per month, accounting for three quarters of the $223 billion in healthcare costs associated with excessive alcohol intake.[14]

Even more alarming, the average number of drinks per binge was eight to nine, leaving medical researchers scrambling to find a new term for these heavy nights out, as their current definition of a binge seemed inadequately low. (Perhaps "double binge" is most fitting!)

In truth, it's easier to over-consume than you realize. The average wine glass has dramatically increased in size over the last decade, which means every glass at your favourite restaurant is worth almost *two* units in the aforementioned studies. Therefore, having two tall glasses of wine for a woman means you are classified as having a binge night out. For the guys, having one beer before your meal followed by two glasses during dinner means a binge night, as well.

Why is binge drinking bad for your health? Consuming too much alcohol in one sitting wreaks havoc on your liver, one of the few organs that helps to control blood sugar levels. It sends your blood sugar levels sky high, leading to poor insulin function and weight gain. Adults aged 18-34 are most likely to have the biggest binges, while surprisingly *adults over 65* had the *most binges* per month.

Try to reduce your intake or add one glass of water between every glass of alcohol to slow your intake. Finally, do NOT drink on an empty stomach, as this will exacerbate the blood sugar swings.

IV. THE BENEFITS—LOW-CARB DIETS VS. HIGH-CARB DIETS

The total amount of carbs you should consume depends on your level of health, genetics and your current goals (weight loss and performance). If you are active and a healthy weight, then you will need greater amounts of carbohydrates to sustain your lifestyle. If you are overweight and sedentary, limiting your carb intake will help to support weight loss and fend off inflammation and chronic diseases.

Low-Carb Diet and Weight Loss

If weight loss is your goal, reducing your carbohydrate intake should be your primary target. The research is clear that carbohydrates have the most dramatic impact on blood sugar and insulin levels. If your insulin levels are elevated, your primary fat burning hormone (hormone sensitive lipase) will be turned "off," preventing you from losing weight. So what is the solution? The ketogenic diet.

A *ketogenic diet* refers to a very low carbohydrate, high protein and high fat diet. Typically, this would mean equal or less than 50g of carbohydrates daily (a simple *low-carb* diet typically contains equal or less than 100g). Over the past decade, the ketogenic diet has gained tremendous momentum because of its ability to promote healthy loss of fat mass, while sparing precious muscle mass and improving overall health. (No fad diet required!)

Does this diet really work? Well, the current research is revealing the overwhelming effectiveness of a ketogenic diet for weight loss. For example, a recent study in the *British Journal of Nutrition* showed that those people adopting a very low-carb diet had significant reductions in bodyweight, as well as lower triglycerides and improved good HDL cholesterol.[5] Every month, we see further studies indicating the effectiveness of a ketogenic diet in reducing body-fat and improving health. You've got nothing to lose except unwanted fat!

Low-Carb Diets and Better Blood Pressure

The studies supporting the use of ketogenic diets for weight loss and improving overall health are growing by the day. In Spain, a recent study of obese people adopting a very low-carb diet (less than 50g per day) showed dramatic improvements in blood pressure, reducing systolic levels by almost 20mmHg and diastolic levels by over 10mmHg.[6] These are really incredible improvements!

Low-Carb Diet and Better Heart Health

The effects of a low-carb diet are beneficial even for those already taking medications related to heart health. In patients already taking statin drugs, six weeks of very low-carb dieting (less than 50g) resulted in reduction in blood pressure, triglycerides, inflammation and improvements in insulin sensitivity.[7] These results are very impressive. Patients instructed to take statins by their doctors to reduce their risk of heart attack or stroke will see increased benefits from a very low-carb dietary approach.

Low-Carb Diet and Better Brain Function

Many health experts now believe there is a strong connection between chronically elevated blood sugar levels, brain deterioration and the development of dementia and Alzheimer's disease. The prestigious *New England Journal of Medicine* recently published an article linking elevated blood sugar levels (hemoglobin A1c or HA1c, a marker for your three-month average blood sugars) and increased risk of developing dementia. The researchers followed 2,000 people for almost seven years and found that elevated HA1c levels correlated strongly with brain deterioration and increased risk of developing dementia.[8]

The most alarming finding was that these patients were NOT even diabetic; their blood sugar levels were *within the normal range!* Yet those with high normal blood sugar results were still at seven times greater risk of developing dementia. These results show the need to revise our current medical standard of *"healthy"* blood sugar levels.

LOW-CARB DIETS AND ATHLETES

A recent study examined athletes who performed "two-a-day" training sessions and consumed only 40% of their total calories as carbohydrates. Not surprisingly, the results showed that athletes on low-carb diets suffered a decrease in their performance because they did NOT adequately replenish muscle glycogen stores.[9]

Intense training will quickly deplete glycogen stores, greatly limiting your performance during your next training session. If you are training at high intensity and following a low-carb diet, you are treading a fine line. Eventually, you will exhibit signs of overtraining and exhaustion.

Overtraining can be experienced in the short term or long term. Short-term symptoms include fatigue during training, poor recovery and extended delayed onset muscle soreness (DOMS). Long-term symptoms of overtraining are reduced time to fatigue, reduced strength levels and increased muscular weakness.

In China (2009), a study examined the effects of high-glycemic meals after exercise on performance in runners. The results showed athletes consuming high-GI meals 90 minutes post-training had significantly improved work capacity during their subsequent run four hours later.[10] This is extremely important for endurance athletes and anyone training at high intensity because high-GI foods are critical for refilling your glycogen stores and ensuring your best performance in training or on race day (more to come in Chapter 10—Upgrade Your Performance).

V. THE PALEO PROJECT—CARB SOLUTIONS

You should aim to consume *clean carbs* (gluten-free) as a regular part of a Modern Paleo diet in accordance with your goals. Figure 3.4 gives you a list of healthy, gluten-free carbs. As a general rule, men should aim to consume a carb serving size equal to two cupped hands per meal, while women should aim for one cupped hand per meal.[15] Your carb intake should be derived from a variety of whole foods to ensure a full spectrum of vitamins, minerals and nutrients.

For weight loss or to improve poor health, you should reduce your carb intake (the more overweight, the more restricted), while performance athletes need to achieve an optimal dose to maximize performance and recovery.

SUMMARY OF HEALTHY 'CLEAN' CARBS			
Roots & Tubers	**Pseudo–Cereals**	**Cereal Grains**	**Veggies & Fruits**
Sweet Potatoes	Quinoa	Brown Rice	Unlimited veggies
Yams	Amaranth	Wild Rice	Fruits in moderation.
Yucca	Buckwheat	Oats	*(All types allowed)*
Jicama		Millet	
Plantains			
Turnips			
Parsnips			
Rutabaga			
Beets			
Carrots			

Figure 3.4. Summary of Healthy "Clean" Carbs

Figure 3.5 is a *Carb Solutions Action Plan*. Review the list of objectives and make sure you are incorporating all the points listed. You've now completed Section I (Nutrition) and have all the tools you need to build a Modern Paleo diet, the foundation of *The Paleo Project*. If this seems like a major shift for you, start with changing just one meal per day (start with breakfast) and then move on to lunch. If you are more comfortable with a Paleo approach or eager to see significant and lasting change, then dive right in!

CARB SOLUTIONS ACTION PLAN

1. Consume a wide range of gluten-free carbs
- 2 'cupped hands' for men; 1 'cupped hand' for women at every meal.

2. Consume unlimited veggies, eat fruit in moderation
- Also, eat a variety of root vegetables, tubers and broadleaf plants.

3. Limit juices, candies, sugars and sweets
- Limit your intake of HFCS, artificial and processed sweeteners.

4. Limit your alcohol consumption
- Ideally, aim for no more than 1-2 alcoholic drinks per day, 2-3 times weekly. If weight loss is your goal, eliminate alcohol completely.

Figure 3.5. Carb Solutions Action Plan

Listed below are various options for increasing your "clean" carbs intake through the day. Remember, men should aim to consume a carb serving size equal to two cupped hands per meal, while women should aim for one cupped hand per meal. If weight loss or improving poor health is your goal, I'll outline in Chapter 9 how to tailor your carb intake to achieve the best results. If performance is your primary goal, I'll discuss in Chapter 10 how you can personalize your carb intake to meet your goals.

Breakfast Options

1. Eggs (4-6 for men; 2-4 for women) + avocado + *oats*

2. Protein shake (30-40g) + coconut oil + *banana + handful of spinach*

3. Chicken breast (or any other meat) + grass-fed butter + *yams*

4. Vegetarian option – Full-fat plain yogurt (1 cup) + *berries*

Snacks (AM)

- Walnuts (approximately 7-8 nuts) + *carrots*

- Full-fat yogurt (approximately 1 cup) + *apple*

Lunch Options

1. Salmon fillet + avocado + *quinoa*

2. Grass-fed beef + macadamia oil + *yucca chips*

3. Turkey breast + olive oil + *short-grain brown rice*

4. Vegetarian Option – Tempeh + *short-grain brown rice*

Snacks (PM)

- Macadamia nuts (approximately 7-8 nuts) + *cherry tomatoes*

- Kefir (approximately 1 cup) + *berries*

Dinner Options

1. Pork + red palm oil + *plantains*

2. Black cod + olive oil + *root vegetable medley*

3. Bison + ghee + *jicama*

4. Vegetarian Option – Yellow Lentils + *quinoa*

SECTION II

Hacking Your Health

"Health is not simply the absence of disease."
~Linus Pauling PhD, Nobel Prize Winner

In Section I, I debunked common myths about proteins, fats and carbs and gave you the framework for integrating a Modern Paleo diet in your life. For some, this will be a gradual process. For others, you will jump in with both feet. Either way, upgrading your diet with more Paleo-friendly meals will improve your health by optimizing your intake of essential nutrients, vitamins and minerals.

In Section II, I'll discuss how important systems of the body—digestion, immunity, inflammation and hormones (cortisol and insulin)—all affect your quest for better health, weight loss and superior performance at work or in the gym.

This is where things get really interesting. We are conditioned to wait for sickness or disease to set in before visiting a doctor but I'll show you how to play detective and investigate your own health. You will learn how to "hack your health" or assess how well your body is functioning.

The traditional medical approach focuses on correcting symptoms and while this is excellent for acute and emergency care, it hasn't shown as much success with chronic conditions. If your house were on fire, you wouldn't be worried about putting out the smoke (the symptoms)— you would be focused entirely on putting out the fire (the root cause)!

A medical approach that focuses on correcting the root causes of illness or health imbalances (rather than just the symptoms) is called functional medicine. This is a 21st century approach to healthcare and wellness that is gaining momentum with expert doctors, researchers and wellness practitioners.

Functional testing should be a fundamental part of how you look after your health. If key systems of your body are not running smoothly, your ability to upgrade your health, lose weight and improve performance will suffer. If you've reached a plateau in your quest to shed body fat or set a new personal best, pay special attention to this section. People are often unaware they have a digestive, immune or hormonal imbalance. Just as you evaluate your business or finances, bring the same rigour to evaluating your health. Fix minor problems before they become major problems.

In the next five chapters, you will *hack your health* by taking a series of *Self-Assessments*. In the same way a pilot would ensure that all systems in the plane are running optimally before taking off, you are going to make sure all your systems are running effectively. Dysfunctions in any of these systems—digestion, immunity, inflammation and key hormones cortisol and insulin—will derail your health, weight loss and performance progress. Just like your core muscles are critical for optimal movement, these systems are the core of the *Paleo Project Pyramid* (Figure C), and they must be strong for you to have the best chance at success.

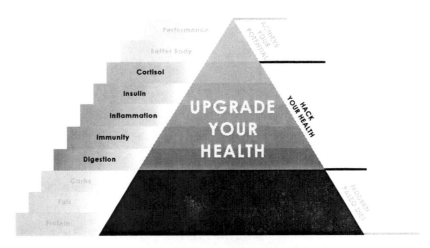

Figure C. The Paleo Project Pyramid—Section II

A word of advice—don't try and implement all the solutions in Section II at once. Simply take it one chapter at a time. If you pass the *self-assessment*, implement the preventative strategies and move on to the next chapter. If you do not pass, continue to support that system while pursuing your quest for weight loss or better performance (you will choose which direction to go in Section III). You are about to upgrade your health and change your body for the long term. Take the plunge. You'll quickly see and feel the difference!

CHAPTER 4

DIGESTION—The Athlete's Engine

Most people assume everything they eat gets broken down and absorbed with 100% efficiency by their digestive system. Unfortunately, this is not always the case. Your digestive system is heavily taxed by chronic stress, intense training, poor food choices, weight gain, lack of sleep, prescription medications, alcohol and chronic infections. These factors quickly derail your digestion and subsequently your quest for better health, a better body and better performance.

In short, the digestive system is your *engine* and it must be running on all cylinders for you to look and perform at your best!

You'd be surprised how many people think it's normal to fart all day or spend a good half hour in the bathroom before being able to have a bowel movement. Many clients who come to see me have spent years dealing with acid reflux through a constant supply of over-the-counter antacids. Digestive issues have become the norm.

We don't like to talk about it, smell it or look at it. Yet what is expelled from our bodies at the end of the digestive process is a clear indicator of our digestive health. It's my goal to make you more aware of how your digestive system is performing. Yes, this can be uncomfortable, but no more uncomfortable than the bout of constipation or acid reflux that you face should you continue to ignore your digestive health!

Digestion is at the base of the *Paleo Project Pyramid* because if things go wrong here, it can easily lead to dysfunctional immunity, inflammation and hormonal imbalance. Do you suffer from an undiagnosed leaky gut that is heavily taxing your immunity? Are you taking stomach acid lowering medications for a heartburn problem that may be *caused* by low stomach acidity? Is digestive weakness causing your low energy levels, sugar cravings, joint pain or slow recovery? Just like dominoes, if one goes over, the repercussions are far reaching!

Your health is intricately connected with the health of the *microbiom* of bacteria in your gut. Unfortunately, many of today's food and life-style choices affect these bacteria, shifting the harmonious balance and wreaking havoc on your digestion and general health.

I. BACK TO BASICS—DIGESTIVE SYSTEM 101

How important is the digestive tract? Gut expert *David Leischeid, ND, PhD,* says that you can understand the importance of a bodily system by determining how many resources are directed toward it. The digestive tract makes up only 6% of your total bodyweight but requires 10-20% of the body's energy output, 25% of the heart's cardiac output (at rest) and over 50% of your essential amino acid pool.[1] That is a tremendous amount of resources for a single system of the body, so it must be important.

Your gut works 24/7 and is home to billions upon billions of health-promoting intestinal bacteria. These good gut bacteria are classified as *probiotics* due to their beneficial symbiotic relationship with the body. Supporting the growth of probiotic gut flora has many benefits, including:

- Preventing constipation

- Protecting you from infection

- Fighting inflammation

- Producing key nutrients in the body

The right food choices help to promote the ideal terrain for optimal digestion. Unfortunately, the wrong food choices create an imbalance in your gut, causing an ideal breeding ground for bad bacteria and a whole host of problems.

A Review of Digestion—From Your Mouth to Down South
In Section I, I discussed how proteins, fats and carbs are digested. Let me review the process and put it all together. Before you put the first piece of food into your mouth, the simple aroma of food triggers the salivary glands to produce *amylase and lipase*, the enzymes that kick-start your carbohydrate and fat digestion, respectively. These enzymes carry out their work while you chew each bite, a major reason you should chew your food thoroughly, as your mother always told you!

As the food moves down into your stomach, special cells (parietal cells) begin increasing the acidity of your stomach in preparation for optimal digestion. Like an orchestra in perfect harmony, the production of hydrochloric acid (HCl) in your stomach initiates the conversion of the enzyme *pepsinogen* to *pepsin*, your primary protein-digesting enzyme. The stage is now set for optimal digestion. Your stomach acidity is high and pepsin is activated.[2] This process has evolved over hundreds of thousands of years to enable you to breakdown and absorb your food. Unfortunately, modern living has caused a few kinks in the process (more on this in the section "How Things Go Wrong").

After the food has been churned and mixed in your stomach, it descends into the first section of your small intestine called the duodenum. Amazingly, a whopping 95% of all your nutrients are absorbed here.[1] In the duodenum of your small intestine (upper bowel), *cholecystokinin (CCK)* is produced to help further breakdown fats and proteins, while initiating the formation of another important enzyme called *trypsin*. Trypsin teams up with CCK to continue breaking down proteins into their most basic individual amino acid parts.

These individual amino acids—critical building blocks of your lean muscle, hormones and immune cells—are then absorbed into your bloodstream through the intestinal villi, small finger-like projections that line your gut in order to enhance absorption.[3] Your intestinal microvilli contain vital digestive enzymes—lactase, maltase and sucrase—that break down disaccharides into their most easily absorbable forms. The majority of your carbohydrate digestion takes place in the small intestine and if you are not digesting carbs well, it destroys the balance of good and bad gut bacteria (more on this later in the chapter).

The duodenum is a busy intersection for digestion because your pancreas and gallbladder also join in the game. CCK triggers the release of more digestive enzymes—*pancreatic amylase, pancreatice lipase and protolytic enzymes*—from your pancreas that continue to breakdown your carbs, fats and proteins into smaller and smaller pieces. You can see the interplay between the stomach, pancreas and gallbladder in Figure 4.1.

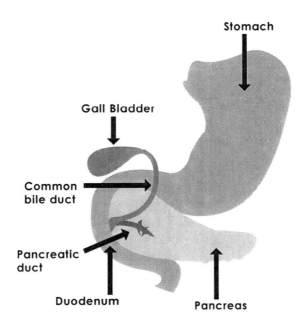

Figure 4.1. The Pancreas and Gallbladder

Your gallbladder is responsible for continuing the breakdown of fats from your meal. It releases bile to help *emulsify* fats into smaller fat droplets, much like your dishwashing detergent breaking up big stains. As the smaller fat droplets travel down to the ileum (the final segment of your small intestine), they are packaged into compact bundles called *chylomicrons* that travel through your lymphatic system to your liver. This process is intricate and complex. These organs work together to digest and absorb your last meal.

After all the nutrients have been absorbed, the remaining food bolus travels down to the large intestine (lower bowel). Your food will spend about 16 hours in your lower bowel, extracting any remaining water from the food and absorbing vitamins that are produced by the trillions of bacteria feeding off the waste matter. Vitamins B1, B2, B12, biotin and K are all produced in considerable quantities in the large intestine by good gut bacteria. The large intestine, shown in Figure 4.2, is home to some 700 different species of bacteria, with *bacteroides* and *bifidobacterium* making up the bulk of the friendly gut microflora.

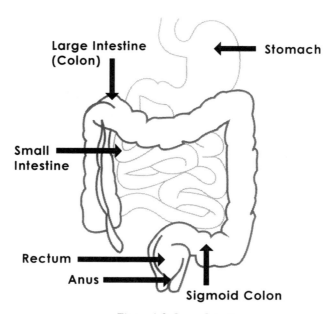

Figure 4.2. Large Intestine

II. "HOW THINGS GO WRONG"—DIGESTIVE DYSFUNCTION

Three out of every five patients I see have some form of digestive dysfunction. It can be so troublesome (persistent gas, bloating and abdominal discomfort) that patients are desperate for relief. On the other hand, it can be as subtle as persistent fatigue, poor immunity, joint pain or low mood that people don't recognize the connection with their gut. The increasing prevalence of sugars and processed foods, the use of genetically modified foods (GMOs), the overuse of antibiotics and painkillers, higher stress levels, eating on the run and inactivity all contribute to poor gut health. I'll discuss the top four scenarios I see in clinical practice.

1. Low Stomach Acidity

2. Intestinal Dysbiosis

3. Leaky Gut (Intestinal Hyper-permeability)

4. Painkillers (NSAIDs)

1) Low Stomach Acidity

Did you know that *low* stomach acidity is a very common condition? It's seen every day in clinical practice and has ripple effects throughout your body. Your stomach is at the top of the digestive chain, so if it's not breaking down your food due to low stomach acid, it will compromise your ability to absorb key nutrients and throw off the balance of good bacteria in your gut.

One of the most common digestive problems is gastro-esophageal reflux disease (GERD), commonly known as heartburn or acid reflux. Typically diagnosed by your doctor, the drugs prescribed to treat GERD top $15 billion a year, making heartburn drugs one of the most prescribed (and profitable) on the market.

Pharmaceutical companies have convinced us that heartburn is the result of excessive stomach acid production, overflowing up into your throat and leading to the unpleasant symptoms of heartburn. Is this really true? Does the science support this theory? While the prescriptions handed out for heartburn increase as people get older, the science tells us that your stomach acidity levels actually *decrease* as you age.[4]

You may be asking yourself, "If this is true, why do I feel better when I take antacids or my heartburn medications?" Well, the symptoms of irritation in your esophagus are indeed caused by acid, but not excessive acid. It's merely the fact that stomach acid is in the *wrong place* that leads to your symptoms. Remember, any amount of acid in your throat will lead to heartburn or pain.

So what is the real cause of heartburn? It's actually quite simple: increased intra-abdominal pressure (IAP). Renowned microbiologist Dr. Norm Robillard has uncovered that the build-up of bad gut bacteria in your small intestine leads to excessive production of gas and, as a result, increased intra-abdominal pressure.

This pressure forces your stomach contents up into your throat, leading to heartburn. This condition is called small intestine bacterial overgrowth (SIBO), and Dr. Robillard believes it is chiefly due to *low stomach acid* (yes, *low* acidity) and maldigestion of carbohydrates.[5]

Most people are erroneously diagnosed with excessive stomach acid and treated with stomach acid lowering drugs. It's common for patients to stay on heartburn drugs for the rest of their lives; however, the drug manufacturers' *own instructions* state they should only be taken in the *short term*. Long-term use leads to major reductions in stomach acidity, nutrient deficiencies and poor protein digestion. Remember, the heartburn drugs only address the symptoms, not the cause.

Optimal stomach acidity is crucial for inhibiting small intestinal bacterial overgrowth (SIBO). Your normal resting level of stomach acidity (measured in pH scale) is a pH of approximately 3. At this optimal pH or acidity, invading bacteria and viruses (picked up from food, drink or the air you breathe) survive in your stomach for approximately 10-15 minutes. The problem starts when stomach acid levels decline (pH increases), allowing bacteria to make it past your stomach acid defences unharmed and into your small intestine.

As these bacteria build up in your small intestine, they begin feeding off ingested carbohydrates in order to grow. If your stomach acid levels are normal, these carbohydrates would have been broken down before entering your gut and the microbes would starve. But, when stomach acidity is low, these poorly digested carbs provide a bountiful buffet for bad bacteria to grow rapidly, leading to small intestine bacterial overgrowth (SIBO). This overgrowth of bacteria produces the excessive hydrogen gas that leads to gas, bloating and heartburn (GERD). *Note:* If you are overweight, bacterial overgrowth or SIBO is more likely due to the overconsumption of sugars and carbohydrates.

Symptoms of Low Stomach Acidity

You don't have to have heartburn or GERD to suffer from low stomach acid or hypochlorhydria—the medical term for a deficiency of hydrochloric acid (HCl) in the stomach. How do you know if you have hypochlorhydria? Common symptoms include the following:

- Belching after eating

- Bloating

- Flatulence immediately after meals

- Feeling of fullness

- Iron deficiency

- Nausea after taking supplements

- White spots or vertical ridges on your nails

- Inability to absorb minerals

- Undigested food in your stool

- Difficulty digesting high protein meals

- Pernicious anemia (low B12)[6]

If any of these symptoms sound familiar, there is a good chance you are deficient in stomach acid.

Causes of Low Stomach Acid

How do you develop low stomach acidity? The most common cause of hypochlorhydria is a bacterial *h.pylori* infection, a frequent finding in clinical practice (one in two people have an *h. pylori* infection by the age of 80!) Other common causes include elevated stress levels (mental or physical), zinc deficiency, high alcohol intake, chronic NSAID (non-steroidal anti-inflammatory drugs) and heartburn drugs.[1] Omeprazole is the generic name for *Prilosec*, the most commonly prescribed proton-pump inhibitor (PPI) or drugs that lower stomach acidity. Ironically, patients taking omeprazole are 50% more likely to develop bacterial overgrowth in the stomach or small intestine (SIBO), further exacerbating their heartburn.[7]

2) Intestinal Dysbiosis

Humans have evolved over millions of years *alongside* the beneficial bacteria that live inside and outside your body. In fact, we've evolved hand-in-hand with these "old friends" who play a tremendous role in shaping our health and wellbeing. Who are these old friends? Your gut is home to hundreds of billions of good bacteria with whom we've evolved over millennia and who've shaped the development of our digestive and immune systems.

Did you know that you have more bacteria in your gut than you have cells in your entire body combined! The *Old Friends Hypothesis* was developed by scientific researchers to describe how our evolution has proceeded in unison with these beneficial bacteria that play a key role in shaping our health. These friendly probiotic bacteria help to assimilate nutrients, produce essential vitamins, balance immune function, cool inflammation and assist in detoxification. It's a beneficial *symbiotic relationship* between you and these billions of good bacterial microflora.

Your health is intricately connected with the health of the bacterial *microbiom* in your gut. Unfortunately, many of today's food and lifestyle choices affect these bacteria, shifting the harmonious balance and compromising your digestive and immune systems.

Intestinal dysbiosis is the term used to describe an imbalance of pathogenic bad to good gut bacteria. Dysbiosis damages the integrity of your gut wall and negatively impacts weight gain, mood, inflammation and hormonal balance.

Symptoms of Dysbiosis

If you have intestinal dysbiosis, you may experience some of the following symptoms: gas, bloating, cramps, fatigue, food allergies, irritable bowel syndrome (IBS), constipation or loose stools. Check out the summary in Figure 4.3. Alternatively, you may have intestinal dysbiosis and not experience any symptoms at all! Clinical studies show that significant gut damage can occur due to intestinal dysbiosis without necessarily experiencing external symptoms.[8] That's right—your gut may have a problem and you are completely unaware!

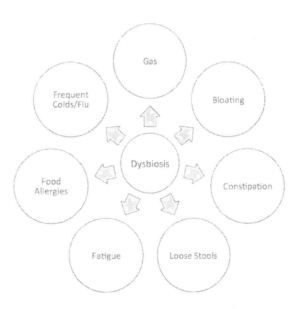

Figure 4.3. Common Symptoms of Intestinal Dysbiosis

Causes of Dysbiosis

How does bad gut bacteria proliferate and cause dysbiosis? There are many aggravating factors including low stomach acid, high stress, diets high in refined sugar, alcohol, processed carbohydrates, too much coffee, unhealthy fats and the overuse of antibiotics.[9]

The frequent use of antibiotics is a major cause of dysbiosis. While antibiotics kill off foreign invading bacteria, they also kill off all of your good gut bacteria, setting the stage for dysbiosis. The two most common good gut bacteria, *Lactobacillus acidophilus and bifidobacterium* are dramatically reduced when you take antibiotics. After a course of antibiotics, opportunistic pathogens such as *E. Coli* and *Candida albicans* can quickly take root.

The reality is that antibiotics are over-prescribed to the point where the World Health Organization (WHO) has issued repeated warnings to doctors to reduce antibiotic prescriptions, due to growing concerns about the development of antibiotic-resistant strains of bacteria.[10] Remember, most colds and flu are self-limiting illnesses and will resolve on their own. (In Chapter 5—Immunity, I discuss strategies to improve your immunity).

THE GUT-IMMUNITY CONNECTION

Your digestion is intricately linked with your immune system. Amazingly, 70% of your immune system is located in your gut, forming your body's first line of defence against pathogens or foreign invaders (bacteria, viruses, parasites, etc.). This is extremely important because bacteria must latch on to your gut membrane and penetrate your cells to cause sickness and disease. Probiotics prevent bad gut bacteria from adhering to your gut cells so they can't attack your body. I'll discuss this in more detail in the next chapter.

3) Leaky Gut

Leaky gut syndrome is the term used to describe a state of *intestinal permeability*, when toxins, microbes, undigested proteins and other large molecules are capable of *passing through your intestinal wall* and making their way into your bloodstream. This leads to a plethora of problems.

Ideally, your gut wall provides a protective barrier that prevents these microbes and molecules from penetrating your bloodstream. Nutrients are absorbed in only one of two ways: through the cells of your gut wall (*transcellular* absorption) or by passing through the tight junctions that keep your intestinal cells closely packed together (*paracellular* absorption). The graphic in Figure 4.4 will help you visualize the process. A leaky gut allows foreign bacteria and molecules to pass through these tight junctions into the bloodstream, triggering a subsequent immune and inflammatory response.

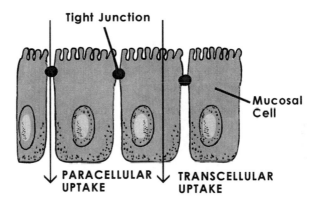

Figure 4.4. Tight Junctions of Gut and Absorption

A leaky gut is the perfect storm for weight gain, poor performance and inadequate recovery. The constant stream of foreign invaders (microbes, toxins and undigested proteins) eventually leads to chronic inflammation and chronic over-activation of your immune system.

In reality, your immune system can cope with a mild influx of foreign molecules or leaky gut. On average, in a fully healthy digestive tract one in every million proteins escapes the digestive process and causes an immune system alarm reaction.[11] In a healthy gut, this will not cause a problem. In a leaky gut, it's a different story.

If you have a leaky gut, your immune system gets flooded with *hundreds of times* this number of *foreign molecules*, which easily pass through your gut wall and cause a major response from your immune system. This excessive immune response leads to chronic inflammation and the free flow of even more undigested food, toxins, unwanted yeasts and bacteria into the bloodstream, shown in Figure 4.5. It becomes a vicious downward cycle. (I discuss this relationship further in Chapter 6—Inflammation).

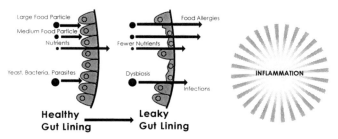

Figure 4.5. Free Passage of Yeasts, Bacteria and Parasites into the Gut

Symptoms of Leaky Gut

You can experience a wide array of symptoms with leaky gut syndrome, including gas and bloating, dysbiosis, abdominal pain, fatigue, chronic joint pain, chronic muscle pain, foggy thinking, compromised immunity and constipation. However, you may not experience any of these symptoms. Leaky gut can be "silent" yet still compromise your health, weight loss and performance.

Causes of Leaky Gut

Common causes of *leaky gut* are stress, the use of NSAIDs, bacterial or viral infections, antibiotics, gluten consumption, toxins and parasites.[12] All of these factors can damage the *tight junctions* that hold your intestinal cells (enterocytes) closely together. As these tight junctions are broken down, the intestinal lining becomes more porous and a leaky gut develops.

For example, the presence of "gram-negative" bacteria in your gut is a common cause of leaky gut. These bad bacteria contain lipopolysaccharides (LPS) on their outer cell membranes, which act as toxins that damage the tight junctions and allow particles to pass freely into your bloodstream. Review the list of common causes of leaky gut in Figure 4.6.

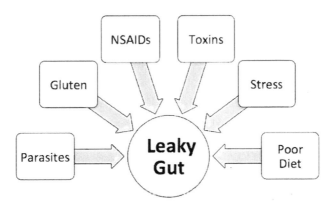

Figure 4.6. Causes of Leaky Gut Syndrome

THE GUT-BRAIN CONNECTION

Busy workdays and high-intensity training can severely impact your digestion. They are both powerful stimuli for your "fight or flight" sympathetic nervous system, which shunts blood away from the digestive organs and towards working muscles during periods of stress (meeting deadlines at work or pushing through a hard workout). This constant sympathetic fight or flight dominance means less time spent in the "rest and digest" mode, the parasympathetic nervous system that rebuilds your body and keeps your digestive system strong. Eventually, this imbalance compromises your digestive function.

4) Painkillers

Non-steroidal anti-inflammatory drugs (NSAIDs) such as ibuprofen (i.e., Advil) and naproxen (i.e., Aleve) are widely used by weekend warriors, professional athletes, desk workers and stay-at-home parents suffering from chronic aches and pains. Doctors and coaches often recommend these over-the-counter NSAID drugs to treat muscular pain and soft tissue injuries and to control inflammation. Although these drugs stop pain, NSAIDs have serious negative effects on your body. Unfortunately, there is no biochemical free lunch in this world!

New research shows that the *chronic use of NSAIDs is a direct cause of intestinal permeability* or leaky gut syndrome.[13, 14] This means that by taking NSAIDs in the long term, you will actually cause leaky gut and chronic inflammation due to the damaging effects on your gut wall.[15]

The problems with taking NSAIDs long term don't end there. They actually *inhibit your ability to build new cartilage and soft tissue.*[15] That's right, the drug prescribed by your doctor to help with joint pain will actually weaken your soft tissue in the long term. Finally, NSAIDs are damaging to your stomach, a major reason why they are a *leading cause of stomach ulcers.*

In spite of this scientific evidence, NSAIDs are the primary medication prescribed to treat injuries and pain syndromes, yet they are responsible for over 100,000 hospitalizations annually. It's not the ideal solution for pain and inflammatory support (more on this in Chapter 6—Inflammation). While these drugs can be effective in the short term (1-5 days), long-term use should be avoided completely unless absolutely necessary.

III. THE PALEO PROJECT—DIGESTION PLAN

If your digestive *engine* is not running smoothly, it can take its toll on your ability to lose weight, your performance in the gym (or at work), your recovery after exercise and your ability to fight off colds and flu. Intense training or poor nutrition can quickly lead to intestinal dysbiosis, the overgrowth of bad gut bacteria and subsequently intestinal damage and leaky gut.

STEP A: SELF-ASSESSMENT

Complete the three *digestion* self-assessments—*Stomach Acidity, Dysbiosis, and Leaky Gut*—below to evaluate your current state of digestive health. Each Yes answer equals a score of 1. Calculate your total score in the boxes below to determine your areas of weakness.

STOMACH ACIDITY SELF-ASSESSMENT

- Do you frequently burp after meals?

- Do you have a low appetite in the morning?

- Are your fingernails weak or have vertical ridges?

- Do you have undigested food in your stool?

- Are you iron deficient?

- Do you have chronic infections (candida or parasites)?

- Do you have any food allergies?

- Do you experience bloating or gas?

- Have you been diagnosed with gastro-esophageal reflux disease (GERD)?

- Have you regularly taken proton pump inhibitors (acid blockers) or antacids?

STEP A: SELF-ASSESSMENT		STEP B: HACK YOUR HEALTH	STEP C: STOMACH ACIDITY SOLUTIONS		
Grade	Score	Lab Testing	Level 1 (Diet)	Level 2 (Bitters)	Level 3 (HCl + Pepsin)
Pass	0-1	n/a	✔	n/a	n/a
Possible Deficiency	2-4	✔	✔	✔	n/a
Support Required	5+	✔	✔	✔	✔

Figure 4.7. Stomach Acidity Action Plan

DYSBIOSIS SELF-ASSESSMENT

- Do you experience gas, bloating or abdominal discomfort?

- Have you been diagnosed with irritable bowel syndrome (IBS)?

- Do you regularly have loose stools?

- Do you regularly miss days (stool)?

- Do you have mucous or blood in the stool?

- Do you experience brain fog?

- Do you experience sinus congestion?

- Are you intolerant to carbohydrates?

- Do you regularly use antacids?

- Have you used antibiotics in the last year?

STEP A: SELF-ASSESSMENT		STEP B: HACK YOUR HEALTH	STEP C: DYSBIOSIS SOLUTIONS		
Grade	**Score**	**Lab Testing**	**Level 1** (Diet)	**Level 2** (Probiotics)	**Level 3** (Berberine)
Pass	0-1	n/a	✔	n/a	n/a
Possible Deficiency	2-4	✔	✔	✔	n/a
Support Required	5+	✔	✔	✔	✔

Figure 4.8. Dysbiosis Action Plan

LEAKY GUT SELF-ASSESSMENT

- Did the dysbiosis self-assessment reveal a possible or likely result?

- Do you have many food allergies?

- Do you have an autoimmune condition?

STEP A: SELF-ASSESSMENT		STEP B: HACK YOUR HEALTH	STEP C: LEAKY GUT SOLUTIONS		
Grade	**Score**	**Lab Testing**	**Level 1** (Diet)	**Level 2** (Glutamine)	**Level 3** (Quercetin + Zinc)
Pass	0	n/a	✔	n/a	n/a
Possible Deficiency	1	✔	✔	✔	n/a
Support Required	2+	✔	✔	✔	✔

Figure 4.9. Leaky Gut Action Plan

STEP B: HACK YOUR HEALTH (LAB TESTING)

Now that you have identified your areas of digestive weakness, it's time to do more in-depth testing. This step will establish the baseline of your current state of health or dysfunction and can be used to track your progress.

If your scores from Step 1 revealed "possible deficiency" or "support required," read the section that applies to you below. If you passed all the self-assessments, move on to Step C (Digestion Solutions) for preventative solutions.

Lab Testing for Stomach Acidity

Good digestion starts in the stomach. Age, chronic infection, stress and high-intensity training all contribute to low levels of stomach acidity. The most convenient and comfortable method of assessing your stomach acidity is the HCl Challenge test.

The goal of the HCl Challenge test is to assess the current levels of stomach acid that are critical for optimal digestive health *downstream* from the stomach in your small intestine and colon. This protocol involves gradually increasingly your intake of supplemental hydrochloric acid (HCl) + pepsin capsules at mealtime over the course of 4 weeks in order to assess your degree of stomach acidity (see Appendix A for detailed instructions).

One of the most common causes of low stomach acidity is *h. pylori* bacterial infection. These bacteria suppress your natural production of stomach acid. In fact, the majority of people with *h. pylori* infections do *not* experience any overt symptoms. If your *HCl Challenge* score is 5+ or more, then getting assessed for *h. pylori* infection via specific breath or stool testing is recommended.

Note: Zinc levels should also be evaluated with hypochlorhydria because it is crucial for supporting HCl production in the stomach. This can be done via blood testing.

Lab Testing for Dysbiosis and Leaky Gut

The best tool for assessing the functional health of your gut is called the Complete Stool Analysis (CSA). This functional test measures specific markers that reflect how well your digestive engine is functioning, the balance of good and bad bacteria, levels of inflammation, markers of a healthy gut (short-chain fatty acids or SCFA) and important immune parameters critical for optimal gut health. By identifying the area of digestive weakness, you can begin a targeted dietary and supplementation protocol to solve the problem. This test can be run by Doctors Data or Metametrixx labs. (*Note:* Leaky gut can also be assessed using the Lactulose/Mannitol test.)

STEP C: DIGESTION SOLUTIONS

In order to support a healthy digestive system and address your underlying digestive weaknesses, refer to the three action plan summary tables above, *figures 4.7, 4.8* and *4.9*. Once you have determined your required levels of support—based on your self-assessments—use the solutions below to build your personalized plan for improved digestion.

STOMACH ACIDITY SOLUTIONS

Level 1 Solution: Diet

If you scored a "pass" on your *Stomach Acidity* self-assessment, a simple and effective approach to naturally stimulate HCl production is to ingest apple cider vinegar (½ to 1 tablespoon) before meals. To support digestive enzymes, add more fermented foods to your diet such as sauerkraut and fresh pickles. In addition, try using pineapple or papaya as a dessert at the end of your meals to improve digestion because these foods contain the digestive enzymes bromelain and papain, respectively.

To help with the digestion of fats, include foods that support the production of bile (the fat emulsifier) from your liver such as horseradish, daikon radish, dandelion, chicory and bitter greens. Finally, if you experience mild heartburn or GERD, then cooling inflammation in your throat tissue is important. Try using oats, flaxseeds and plantains to soothe the irritation or sip herbal teas such as marshmallow or slippery elm.

Level 2 Solution: Herbal Bitters

If you scored "possible deficiency" on your *Stomach Acidity* self-assessment then adding more robust support for stomach function is advised.
A traditional holistic remedy for naturally increasing stomach acidity
is the use of herbal bitters, such as gentian, ginger, fennel or a formula
called Canadian Bitters. Simply add 1-2ml (10 drops) directly on to
your tongue to help kick-start the digestive process at mealtime.

Level 3 Solution: Betaine Hydrochloride + Pepsin

If you scored "support required" on your *Stomach Acidity* self-assessment
then performing the HCl Challenge is strongly indicated. Perform the
protocol as outlined in Appendix A and, based on the results of your
test, follow this prescription protocol:

If you finished the HCl Challenge taking three capsules or less, then
discontinue the HCl supplementation after you've finished the bottle,
and implement the Level 2 protocol for continual support.

If you finished the challenge taking four capsules or more, there is
likely more to the story than just low stomach acidity. You may

have a deficiency of other key digestive enzymes (see *Appendix A—HCl Challenge*).

DYSBIOSIS SOLUTIONS

Level 1 Solution: Diet

If you scored a "pass" on your *Dysbiosis* self-assessment, it's important to maintain healthy gut microflora over the long run by integrating more healthy eating habits. To prevent dysbiosis from rearing its ugly head, follow these quick tips:

Remove Aggravating Foods

In order to maintain a healthy intestinal microflora (and avoid falling back into the same old patterns), it is crucial for you to avoid foods that stimulate the growth of bad gut bacteria. Sugars, simple and white carbs, and breads are the preferred foods for harmful bacteria, so be sure to remove these from your diet. These foods will lead to gas and bloating and damage the lining of your gut wall. A Modern Paleo diet is free of all these foods.

Other common foods that disrupt gut function are *fructose* (from HFCS, sweeteners and processed foods), *lactose* (from dairy products) and *gluten* (from breads and processed foods). Incorporating more Modern Paleo meals into your diet will naturally limit these foods. Remember, chemical sweeteners such as Sucralose or other sugar alcohols destroy bacterial flora, so try and steer clear of those as well. To curb your sweet tooth try honey, maple syrup, molasses or cane sugar in moderation.

Introduce Fermented Foods

Next, adding in naturally occurring probiotics from *fermented foods* such as plain yogurt, kefir, sauerkraut, kimchi, tamari sauce, natto miso and kombucha tea is a great way to support optimal gut microflora in the long term. If you react to dairy, try goats' milk or sheep's milk yogurt, or coconut milk yogurt. In addition, *green tea* has been shown to increase the number of beneficial gut bacteria due to the presence of polyphenols. By including these Modern Paleo staples regularly in your diet, you will be able to maintain a healthy gut flora through diet alone.

Add More Fibre and Resistant Starch

Adding natural soluble fibre sources to your diet, particularly *pectins* found in apples, apricots, cherries, carrots, oranges and berries will go a long way in supporting healthy gut microflora.[16] Probiotics love fibre! Soluble fibre improves *transit time*, a medical term for the length of time between bowel movements. The less frequent your bowel movements, the greater the likelihood of bacterial overgrowth and poor health. Fibre also supports healthy blood sugar levels and reduces your risk of cardiovascular disease.[17] If you struggle with sluggish bowels, adding a soluble fibre supplement can be beneficial in the short term while you re-establish normal gut motility.

Resistant starch (RS) is a new classification of carbohydrate that does not get fully digested and absorbed in the small intestine, thus passing into the large intestine relatively intact to serve as a food source for your good gut bacteria. In effect, RS carbs are *resistant* to digestion. New research is uncovering the benefits of resistant starch foods on your digestion and health. By including more of these foods in your diet, you'll be providing your gut microflora with all the nourishment they need to remain vibrant and healthy.

The three main types of resistant starches include:

- RS1 – beans, grains, seeds (starch bound by indigestible cell walls)

- RS2 – potatoes, plantains (starch naturally indigestible in raw state)

- RS3 – grains, potatoes, beans (retrograde starch, cooked and then cooled)

Level 2 Solution: Probiotics

If you scored "possible deficiency" on your *Dysbiosis* self-assessment, then adding a probiotic supplement will be highly beneficial for you.

Lactobacilli and *bifidobacterium* are the predominant gut bacteria found in the intestinal tract and play key roles in assisting the breakdown of proteins and carbohydrates, synthesizing vitamins and fatty acids, boosting immune function and converting flavonoids into anti-inflammatory factors. The lack of fermented foods in the typical Western diet means probiotic supplementation benefits almost everyone. Clinical studies show that probiotic supplementation reduces the bloating associated with bowel disorders, as well as supporting optimal gastric health by inhibiting inflammation caused by bacterial infections (most commonly *H. pylori*).[18, 19]

In addition, probiotics exert a potent anti-inflammatory effect on the body, helping to mitigate excessive inflammation from training, weight gain, and injury (more on inflammation in Chapter 5—Immunity and Chapter 6—Inflammation).[20] Be sure to supplement with probiotics that include *fructo-oligosaccharides* (FOS) because they stimulate the growth of healthy gut bacteria (what the probiotics like to eat).[21] Another great benefit of FOS is its ability to improve mineral absorption such as magnesium, zinc, calcium and iron that are crucial for performance, weight loss and optimal health. Get your natural FOS dose in the following whole foods: onions, chicory, garlic, asparagus, banana and artichoke.

Probiotics should be taken with food in divided doses, one to three times daily, depending on the severity of your dysbiosis. Each capsule should contain at least 10 billion bacterial cells for optimal therapeutic benefit. New research also shows that soil-based probiotic organisms (SBOs) are highly effective for repopulating the gut microflora, my favourite choice is Prescript-Assist.

Level 3 Solution: Berberine

If you scored "support required" on your *Dysbiosis* self-assessment, it's highly likely you have a build-up of bad gut bacteria. Therefore, performing a Complete Stool Analysis (CSA) test is highly recommended. This test will help you identify the exact strains of bacteria, yeasts or parasites that have penetrated your defences.

Dysbiosis is much more common than you think. In order to kill off these bugs, you must use a powerful anti-microbial agent: the medicinal herb *goldenseal* fits the bill. Described as "king of the mucous membranes" in herbal medicine texts, goldenseal contains a powerful chemical called berberine, which acts as a potent anti-microbial agent to clear out harmful bacteria, yeasts and parasites from the gut.[22]

Why not just use antibiotics? First, while they do kill the bad bacteria, they also kill your good gut bacteria, leaving you more prone to dysbiosis and future infection (one-step forward, two-steps back). Next, antibiotics deal only with bacterial infections, not yeasts and parasites. By using an herbal antimicrobial, you address all types of pathogens while getting additional immune and blood sugar support. However, be sure to consume adequate amounts of water when taking berberine because it is mildly dehydrating to the body.

The dose of berberine is 200-300mg, two to three times daily away from food. Make sure to take this for four to eight weeks. (*Note:* If taking for more than eight weeks, consult a naturopathic doctor or herbalist.)

LEAKY GUT SOLUTIONS
Level 1 Solution: Coconut Oil and Ghee
Increasing your intake of healthy saturated fats via coconut oil and clarified butter (ghee) is the ideal way to provide the important nutrients that keep your gut wall strong. Try adding coconut oil (1-4 tbsp daily) to your morning oats, protein shakes, as a dip with apples (or fruit), or use it to stir-fry vegetables. Use ghee when cooking vegetables or frying your eggs for breakfast, or simply add on top of veggies at dinnertime. For more scientific information on the benefits of coconut oil and ghee, refer to Chapter 2—Fats.

Level 2 Solution: Glutamine

Glutamine is a key amino acid for rebuilding the integrity of your gut wall. Your levels decrease dramatically (up to 50%) when training intensely or at times of stress. The ideal dose of glutamine is 0.2g/kg bodyweight, which can be taken in divided doses after training and/ or before bed.[23, 24] For example, a 200lb male would consume 18g daily, whereas a 145lb female would consume 13g daily.

Level 3 Solution: Quercetin and Zinc

A naturally occurring bioflavonoid, quercetin supports optimal gastro-intestinal health in several ways. First, it is a strong antioxidant that prevents the oxidation of the healthy fats you eat (or should be eating!).[25] Remember, your GI tract has an increased exposure to oxidative stress due to its lower pH; therefore, quercetin can provide added protection to the fatty cell walls of your gut. Second, quercetin prevents the depletion of glutathione from your intestinal cells, thereby protecting them from toxic free-radical damage.[26] (Vitamin C improves the ability of quercetin to do so.) Finally, it prevents the breakdown of key immune cells (mast cells) that would normally release histamine leading to damage of the intestinal gut lining.[27] A dose of 500mg of quercetin three times daily will support optimal intestinal integrity and help to reverse your leaky gut.

Zinc plays a key role in digestion and maintaining gut integrity. It has been shown to be extremely useful in solving leaky gut, as studies show significant improvements in intestinal barrier function and reductions in permeability with supplementation.[28] Zinc helps to prevent leaky gut by supporting the production of HCl in your stomach. A dose of 30-60mg of zinc at bedtime will support optimal gut health.

CASE STUDY—DIGESTION

Forty-two year old Carlos came to me complaining of serious fatigue and worsening insomnia. The tipping point came when he finished his last race in his worst ever time, despite putting more effort into his training and nutrition. As a busy portfolio manager and active triathlete, he could not afford to be tired throughout the day, struggle to maintain focus at work, and be unable to enjoy family time at home due to exhaustion.

Carlos's health history revealed habitual use of NSAIDs nightly to cope with muscle and joint pain, four to six espressos per day to give him energy, chronic gas and bloating, consistent sugar cravings in the evening and constant waking throughout the night. Based on these symptoms, I decided to run a CSA (Complete Stool Analysis) test to assess his digestive system (the athlete's engine!). Not surprisingly, Carlos's test results, seen in Figure 4.10, revealed significant dysfunctions.

Lab Test	Normal Range	Carlos's Levels	Significance
Bacterial Culture	Expected Flora Bifidobacterium spp. +3-4 Lactobacillus spp. +3-4	Expected Flora Bifidobacterium spp. +1 Lactobacillus spp. +NG	Insufficient 'good' gut bacteria.
	Dysbiotic Flora None present	Dysbiotic Flora Citrobacter braakii +4 Citrobacter farmer +4 Citrobacter freundii +3 Proteus mirabilis +4	Presence of dysbiotic 'bad' gut bacteria
Secretory IgA	50-200	350	High - likely leaky gut
Lactoferrin	Less than 7.3	8.4	High - chronic gut inflammation
Total SCFAs Butyrate SCFA	4-14 0.8-3.8	5 0.8	Low normal – increased likelihood of poor digestive function

Figure 4.10. Summary of Carlos's Lab Test Results

I started Carlos on a protocol to rebalance gut flora, heal his leaky gut and cool inflammation. Carlos stopped his NSAIDs and replaced them with herbal alternatives (more on this in Chapter 6—Inflammation). He reduced his coffee intake to one per day (which was very difficult for the first week, then he noted a major improvement in energy), and added all three levels of the Leaky Gut Solutions in this chapter. Carlos noticed his gas and bloating subsided completely after two weeks, his sugar cravings at night were gone and his energy levels were much better. Carlos's progress translated nicely to his workouts, where his power numbers on the bike were up and, best of all, he achieved his best result of the season in the subsequent race!

CHAPTER 5

IMMUNITY—The Athlete's Armour

Most people pay little attention to their immune system until they get sick. Your immune system is an amazingly complex army of cells constantly battling bacteria, viruses and other pathogens. Your immune system is your armour, protecting you against the many threats your body faces on a daily basis.

Nothing sabotages your performance at work more quickly than missed days due to illness. Being constantly on the go, meeting stressful work deadlines and juggling family and demanding clients can leave you and your immune system running on empty. If you are exercising intensely, training for a competition or pushing yourself to the limit, this also places tremendous stress on your immune system.

You may be saying, "But I never get sick." Well, you don't need to actually be sick to have your immune system compromised because the symptoms express themselves in other ways. Depressed immunity is associated with poor energy, low mood, muscle and joint pain, decreased productivity at work and poor performance or recovery in the gym. These are signs that your immune system may be taxed.

A more efficient immune system means better productivity at work, fewer missed training days and more energy. It also means less chance of catching a nasty cold from your kids or co-workers. If you are striving to achieve weight loss, better performance or to improve your health then maintaining optimal immunity is crucial.

I. BACK TO BASICS—IMMUNE SYSTEM 101

Your immune system consists of a variety of different cells whose job it is to fight off bacteria, viruses, parasites or other foreign invaders that attempt to penetrate your defences. These cells are the *soldiers* that make up your immune system *army* and they are composed of two parts: the innate immune system and the adaptive immune system.

Innate Immune System

The innate immune system and its cells, shown in Figure 5.1, is your body's *first line of defence* against foreign invaders. It is a non-specific reaction to pathogens, meaning it does not target specific bacteria or viruses but triggers a general immune response in the body. Your immune system's first response to an intruder is an inflammatory response, characterized by fever, redness, malaise and pain. Imagine this system is your body's alarm bell, the warning signal that sounds off at the first sign of a threat to your body.

When the alarm goes off, your innate immune systems sends out its *foot soldier* immune cells (neutrophils, macrophages and natural killer (NK) cells) to investigate. Neutrophils make up 50% of your innate immune cell army and are formed from stem cells in your bone marrow. They effectively patrol the body like night watchmen, looking out for the first sign of trouble.

Macrophages are another important cell type in your innate immune system. Their job is to engulf any foreign intruders, like Pacman gobbling up the enemy. They play another important role, sounding off like a bullhorn to tell other innate immune cells that an enemy has been detected and recruit them to join the fight. These include the natural killer (NK) cells, which are immune system snipers that pick off any viruses that penetrate your immune barriers. NK cells are unique because they act quickly and detect stressed cells that have not yet been identified by your immune system.

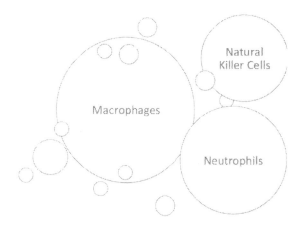

Figure 5.1. Innate Immune System Cells

Adaptive Immune System

If a foreign invader penetrates your body's defences and outsmarts your innate immune system, your highly sophisticated adaptive immune system (shown in Figure 5.2) is called into action. The adaptive immune system differs from innate immunity because it triggers an immune response to a specific antigen (*antigen* is the scientific term for the foreign invaders such as bacteria, viruses, parasites, etc.). This is the equivalent of calling in the army's *special forces* to get the job done. Unlike the foot soldiers of the innate immune system, the adaptive immune system is more highly skilled and designed to track down *specific* foreign invaders and destroy them.

This response doesn't happen as quickly as the innate immune response. It takes longer because your immune system must inform and program the adaptive immune cells to attack the villain. After the immune cells are programmed, your special forces' immune cells are ready to seek and destroy any foreign bacteria or viruses that have penetrated your first line of defence.

What are these special forces adaptive immune cells? Your adaptive immune system consists of T-cells (helper and cytotoxic), B-cells and natural killer (NK) cells (these guys are so good they do double-duty, working for both systems). B-cells are responsible for producing antibodies, which are molecules that tag the foreign invaders so your adaptive immune cells know exactly who to attack. This allows your immune system to differentiate between the bad guys and the good guys (your own cells). After these antibodies attach to intruders, *T-helper* cells produce *cytokines* that kick off an inflammatory reaction, while *cytotoxic T-cells* seek and destroy the enemy.

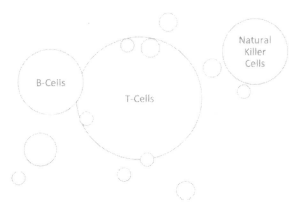

Figure 5.2. Adaptive Immune System Cells

Immune Memory

An important characteristic of your adaptive immune system cells is *memory*. Just like an army sergeant remembering past battles, your adaptive immune cells have a memory of past intruders. This is extremely important because it means that if those cells attack you again in the future, your immune system will remember them and react quickly to destroy them before they cause trouble. This system is the mechanism by which your body acquires resistance to infection or *immunity*. After you are exposed to a particular virus (i.e., chicken pox or malaria) your body has a lifelong immunity against that virus because of your adaptive immune system's memory. Pretty impressive!

Cytokines and Immunity

Your immune system's first response to an intruder is an inflammatory response, which is characterized by fever, redness, malaise and pain. The primary pro-inflammatory molecules associated with this inflammatory response are called *cytokines*. Cytokines are a group of immune system modulators that exert powerful pro- and anti-inflammatory effects on your body.

Digestion and Immunity

In the previous chapter on digestion, I described how intimately your digestive system is connected with your immune system. Amazingly, 70% of your immune system is located in your gut; therefore, any discussion on how to improve immune function inevitably leads back to digestion. If you followed the steps in the previous chapter, you are already well on your way to improving your immunity.

A major building block of the immune system is a protein complex call *secretory immunoglobulin A* (sIgA). It is a mucous layer that lines your gut wall and plays a major role in establishing your body's first line of defence. This barrier protects you from invading bacteria, viruses and undigested proteins.

When your immune system is working efficiently and your stress (physical or mental) is being managed, your sIgA levels will be within normal range. However, intense training, high stress (cortisol) levels, endurance training, intestinal dysbiosis and chronic infections deplete sIgA levels as they use up your precious immune resources over time. Acute infection, autoimmune conditions and food allergies create a heightened immune response, increasing sIgA levels, as shown in Figure 5.3. In general, the greater the digestive dysfunction is, the greater the immune dysfunction (sIgA).

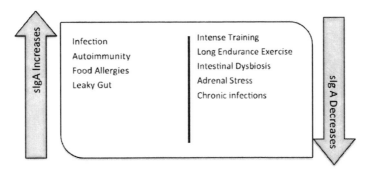

Figure 5.3. Factors Influencing Secretory IgA levels

The right balance of *intestinal microflora* supports a more robust immune system. Probiotics are highly effective at enhancing your adaptive immunity, the "seek and destroy" arm of the immune system. A study in the journal *Clinical and Experimental Immunology* demonstrated that probiotic bacteria stimulate T-cell and natural killer cells, thereby enhancing your immune defence.[1] This type of support is crucial in preventing colds and flu, as well as missed training days or deadlines at work due to illness.

As I discussed in the previous chapter, the modern lifestyle may leave you prone to intestinal dysbiosis and leaky gut. These negative changes in gut flora can quickly derail your immune system. Currently, a growing field of medical research is attempting to identify specific beneficial strains of gut bacteria. Researchers believe there is significant cross talk between probiotic gut bacteria and immune cells that improves both innate and adaptive immunity.[2]

II. HOW THINGS GO WRONG—IMMUNE DYSFUNCTION

How severe was your last cold or flu? Did it knock you out for a week or were you back at work in no time? Did you miss just one training day or did it take you a week or two to recover? Many factors impact your immunity. These things can determine the *severity* and *duration* of your illness, which makes all the difference between being able to go to work or being stuck at home in bed.

1.   Diet

2.   Dehydration

3.   Antibiotics

4.   Food Allergies

5.   Autoimmune Diseases

6.   High Stress

7.   Lack of Sleep

8.   Intense Exercise

1) Diet

Deficiencies in key nutrients limit your immune system's ability to fight off infections. Vitamins D, A and C, along with the mineral zinc and amino acid glutamine are important fuels for your immune system.

Vitamin D

The sun is one of nature's most potent immune boosters, stimulating the production of over 200 antimicrobial peptides that kill off bacteria, viruses and fungi to keep you fit and healthy all year round.[3] If you already have a cold, vitamin D can still help because of its ability to up-regulate T-cell activity, the adaptive immune cells that respond to infections. Research shows that insufficient sunlight actually decreases T-cell production, leaving you more prone to colds and flu.[4]

Vitamin D deficiency is very common in countries with severe winter climates because for many months of the year the sun does not rise high enough in the sky to provide you with your daily vitamin D requirements. Therefore, supplementing with 5,000IU of vitamin D daily from October to March is recommended for most adults. If you are supplementing with higher doses, you should have your levels regularly assessed (25-hydroxy vitamin D). The *Vitamin D Society* recommends adults obtain blood levels between 100–150 mmol/L for optimal health.[5]

Vitamin A

If you frequently get sick or bruise easily then vitamin A deficiency is highly likely. The research shows that vitamin A deficiency impairs mucosal immunity and leaves you more prone to colds and flu.[6] Vitamin A plays a key role in white blood cell production and the activation of T-cells after infection, helping you to fight off infections.

Vitamin A is actually a general term for a group of related compounds: retinal, retinol, retinoic acid. They help to establish mucosal immunity by acting as a protective barrier against intruding pathogens by supporting the cellular integrity of your gut and sinuses.[7]

Vitamin C

It is well established in clinical studies that vitamin C supplementation improves the response of neutrophils and lymphocytes, the front-line soldiers of your innate immune system.[8] If you are training at high intensity or working long hours, increasing your vitamin C intake improves your immunity considerably (as well as reduces cortisol stress hormones).[9] It only takes one cold before an important meeting or competition to sabotage your performance.

Zinc

Zinc is crucial for optimal immunity because it's the primary fuel for your thymus gland, which is responsible for producing the T-cells of your adaptive immune system. Current research shows that zinc supplements reduce both the severity and duration of colds.[10] Typically, athletes are more prone to deficiencies in zinc due to the high intensity and volume of training.

Zinc works synergistically along with vitamin C to enhance your immune system. A recent study of approximately 100 athletes examined the effects of supplementing with a combination of vitamin C and zinc during infections. The authors found a dramatic reduction in both the severity of symptoms and duration of infections in those athletes supplementing with vitamin C and zinc compared to a placebo.[11]

Glutamine
Glutamine is the most abundant amino acid in the body; however, it is quickly depleted from muscle stores after intense exercise. For this reason, it is classified as a *conditionally* essential amino acid, meaning it becomes *essential* under times of stress (physical, mental or emotional). When athletes engage in intense or prolonged exercise their glutamine stores decrease by as much as 50% post-training.[12] As glutamine levels decline, so does your body's ability to fight off infection. Supplementing with glutamine post-training or before bed enhances recovery and reduces susceptibility to colds and flu.[13]

2) Hydration
Water is truly the fluid of life and maintaining proper hydration is a cheap and easy way to improve your immunity. A common mistake is waiting to feel thirsty before drinking water. Unfortunately, by the time you feel thirsty, you are already dehydrated. Studies show that a mere 2% loss in hydration can result in decreased immunity (sIgA) and athletic performance.[14] If you are suffering from a cold or flu, you lose fluids more easily (from your runny nose and hacking cough), further exacerbating possible dehydration.

How do you know if you are well hydrated? A simple and cost-effective strategy to assess for dehydration is to perform a *urinalysis*. This test can measure the *specific gravity* of your urine sample, which reflects your current level of hydration.

3) Too Many Antibiotics
The inappropriate or excessive use of antibiotics weakens your immunity. Antibiotics are designed to eradicate dangerous and harmful bacteria, but they also destroy important immune-regulating probiotic gut bacteria. Lack of beneficial flora in the gut is associated with a poor immune response and increased susceptibility to illness.

The World Health Organization (WHO) has outlined in its position statement that doctors should advise patients not to use antibiotics for mild self-limiting illnesses such colds and flu, which make up the majority of cases. The over-prescription of antibiotics not only damages your gut health but also leads to the development of antibiotic resistant strains of bacteria.

If you must take antibiotics, be sure to include a probiotic supplement taken at different times of the day. Studies show that probiotic supplementation modulates the response of intestinal microflora to the effects of antibiotic therapy, limiting the damage to your good gut bacteria.[15, 16]

4) Food Allergies

Ironically, food may present a serious challenge to your immune system. A *food allergy* refers to a specific immune response (IgE class) after the ingestion of an offending or allergenic food. *Food sensitivity* involves a different arm of your immune system (the IgG class) and therefore elicits a different response. The prevalence of food allergies and food sensitivities has increased markedly over the past decade.

Your gut wall is the last line of defence between you and the outside world. If undigested proteins make it into your bloodstream, your immune system immediately sounds the alarm bell. This signals your immune system to take action, as specific cells tag the foreign intruders so they can be tracked down and destroyed. Unfortunately, your immune system shouldn't be picking fights with foods you are eating (such as peanuts and the gluten in bread). So, what is happening here? Take a closer look.

Food Allergies—IgE

This type of immune reaction is the only example of a true food allergy. The IgE allergic reactions are immediate and intense, commonly triggering outbreaks of redness, hives, watery eyes, swelling or fever. Classic examples of IgE reactions are peanut or shellfish allergies. Testing for IgE food allergies requires a blood draw.

Food Allergies—IgG

Food sensitivities or IgG food allergies typically refer to delayed immune reactions to food. The major difference between IgG and IgE food allergies is that IgG allergies can take several hours or days to manifest in the body and the intensity of the reaction is much less. The IgG antibody sticks itself on to the foreign invader and they pass through the gut wall together. This signals your immune system to seek and destroy the invading particle. Compare the characteristics of each in Figure 5.4.

If your immune system is running smoothly, it will take care of the problem quickly with no repercussions. If your system is overloaded with too many of these foreign substances, it gets overwhelmed and triggers an all-out assault by your immune system. The symptoms of IgG food allergies include fatigue, sluggishness, sinus congestion, dark circles under the eyes, mental fog or lack of focus, gas, bloating and frequent colds and flu.

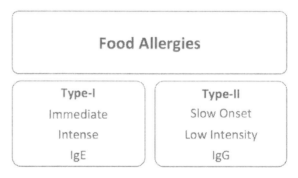

Figure 5.4. Types of Food Allergy

Causes of Food Sensitivity

Digestive dysfunction is the primary reason for food allergies and sensitivities. Poor stomach acidity, intestinal dysbiosis and leaky gut discussed in the previous chapter all contribute to an increased incidence of food allergies. Partially digested food leads to the build-up of opportunistic bad gut bacteria that damage your intestinal wall and microvilli. This micro-trauma allows undigested proteins to penetrate through damaged tight junctions, which are responsible for keeping your gut cells tightly packed together, and into your bloodstream. This contributes to leaky gut and the increased likelihood of food sensitivities or allergies.[17] Other common causes include sluggish liver function, poor pancreatic enzyme production or over-consumption of the same foods.

FOOD INTOLERANCE

A food intolerance is unlike food allergies and sensitivities because it does not involve your immune system. Instead, it refers to a deficiency in a certain enzyme that results in poor digestion or intolerance to a food. For example, people who lack the enzyme lactase have trouble digesting milk and are therefore lactose intolerant.

5) Autoimmune Diseases

Autoimmune diseases are one of the fastest growing illnesses in North America, now affecting more than 24 million people. They develop when your immune system starts attacking your own cells and is no longer able to differentiate between *self* (your body's tissue) and *nonself* (foreign invaders.) Because of this, it treats your own tissue as a foreign invader and mounts an unnecessary attack on your own cells! This damages essential cells, tissues and organs in your body.

Your immune system has two arms—Th1 and Th2. They work together to keep your immune system in balance, shown in Figure 5.5. Imagine two people leaning forward, arms outstretched, holding each other perfectly in place. As long as they maintain their position, they are in perfect balance. However, as soon as one person removes his weight, the other goes tumbling down! This is what happens when your Th1 and Th2 immunity gets out of balance. One system is down-regulated while the other becomes over-active. This is the perfect recipe for developing autoimmune diseases.

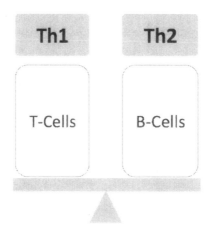

Figure 5.5. Balanced Adaptive Immune System

Autoimmune diseases share another common thread—*chronic inflammation*. Over-active immune responses lead to excessive inflammation that may cause fatigue, joint pain, swelling, abdominal discomfort, gas and bloating, and lack of mental clarity or brain fog. New research suggests that autoimmune diseases and the subsequent immune over-activation is triggered by multiple factors such as stress, infection, heavy-metal exposure and even gluten consumption.

Examples of Th1 dominant autoimmune diseases include multiple sclerosis (MS), Crohn's disease, type-1 diabetes, hashimotos thyroid disease, psoriasis, rheumatoid arthritis and stomach ulcers (*h. pylori* induced). Meanwhile, T2 dominant autoimmune diseases include allergies, asthma, chronic sinusitis, ulcerative colitis, viral infections, lupus and many cancers.

6) High Stress

Stress is intimately connected with your immunity. Elevated stress levels from training, long hours at the office or taking care of the kids depletes important immune cells and inhibits your ability to fight off colds and flu, summarized in Figure 5.6.[18] Blood cortisol levels increase dramatically during exercise and may remain elevated for a long time post-training when engaging in strenuous training, successive bouts of intense training, high-volume endurance exercise or as your competitive season progresses.[19] If your stress levels remain high, it will leave your immune system running on empty.

A study in the *Journal of Strength and Conditioning* followed weightlifters through four training phases as they peaked for a competition. Cortisol and immune parameters were measured throughout the four phases of training. The study found that as the intensity of the training increased, cortisol levels increased and secretory IgA immune levels decreased significantly.[20]

Team sport athletes are affected too. A study in the *European Journal of Applied Physiology* examined the impact of training on immunity in university-level basketball players. Data was taken before, during and after competition as well as throughout their recovery periods. Over the course of a season, researchers found that sIgA levels decreased significantly during the most intense training and competitive phases.[21] The authors concluded that increases in cortisol correlated to decreases in sIgA levels, showing that stress takes a serious toll on your first line of defence immunity. This immune suppression may last for 24 to 72 hours after exercise.

The *Journal of Applied Physiology* examined the immune status of female college volleyball players over the course of a playing season to determine its impact on immunity. The results showed significant reductions in natural killer (NK) cells as the season progressed. Natural killer cells are key immune players that act rapidly in response to viral infections.[22]

Life stress also increases cortisol. For example, mental stress is associated with altered *cortisol rhythm*—your body's natural daily production—that can suppress your immune system (more on this Chapter 8—Cortisol). A recent study showed that employees who do not have clearly defined roles in their job suffer from increased cortisol levels.[23] Also, your perception of a stressful situation or ability to cope with stress greatly affects your cortisol production. Studies show that employees who reported their jobs as stressful tended to have higher cortisol levels during the week (from Monday to Friday) than on weekends.[24] Thus, stress from mental, physical and emotional sources strongly affects your immunity.

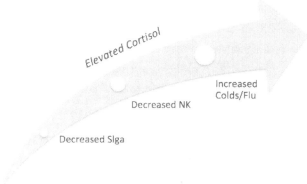

Figure 5.6. Effects of High Cortisol on Immunity

7) Lack of Sleep

Getting adequate sleep is of paramount importance to recover and maintain optimal immune function. Current research shows that factors such as *total sleep quantity* (hours per night) and *sleep quality* (number of awakenings per night) are important factors that affect your immunity.

As your sleep quantity and quality decline, so does your immunity. Not surprisingly, this means an increased risk of more severe colds and flu. In Sweden, a study at the *Karolinska Institute* found that reduced sleep time impaired B-cell, T-cell and natural killer cell function.[25] This finding means that both your innate and adaptive immune systems take a serious hit if you don't get your sleep. If you are working long hours or training for an event such as a marathon, triathlon or CrossFit games, this is a very important point to consider. Make sure to schedule time to get your sleep; nothing derails a podium finish more quickly than being sick on competition day!

8) Intense Training

A single prolonged or high-intensity training bout may suppress your immunity for up to six hours post-training.[1] Repeated bouts of intense training may leave your immune system function depleted for 24-72 hours post-exercise.[19, 26] During this time, your resistance to infection is much lower.

Endurance athletes should pay special attention to this chapter. The latest research shows that excessive aerobic endurance training is more taxing to your immune system than strength or sprint training. This means that endurance athletes are *even more likely* to catch colds or feel fatigued and run down.[2]

Depressed immunity is associated with low energy, depressed mood, muscle and joint pain, decreased productivity at work and poor performance or recovery in the gym. These are all cues that your immune system may be taxed.

III. THE PALEO PROJECT—IMMUNITY PLAN

STEP A: SELF-ASSESSMENTS

Complete the *Immunity* self-assessment and incorporate the corresponding *Immunity Action Plan* in Figure 5.7.

Immunity Self-Assessment

- Do you have a sweet tooth?

- Do you drink less than two litres of water daily?

- Do you have a dry nose and/or throat?

- Do you bruise easily?

- Do you heal slowly from injuries, cuts or sores?

- Do you have low vitamin D levels (or live in northern climate with true winter)?

- Do you regularly experience fatigue, irritability or high stress?

- Are you an endurance athlete?

- Do you NOT supplement with probiotic? (Yes = you do NOT supplement)

- Do you catch more than two colds or flu per year?

- Do you have an autoimmune condition?

- Do you have food allergies?

STEP A: SELF-ASSESSMENT		STEP B: HACK YOUR HEALTH	STEP C: IMMUNITY SOLUTIONS		
Grade	Score	Lab Testing	Level 1 (Diet + Lifestyle)	Level 2 (Herbs + Nutrients)	Level 3 (Colostrum)
Pass	0-2	n/a	✔	n/a	n/a
Possible Deficiency	3-6	✔	✔	✔	n/a
Support Required	7+	✔	✔	✔	✔

Figure 5.7. Immunity Action Plan

Note: If you are acutely sick, implement the *Level 1 Solution* as well as the *Acute Immunity* protocol listed at the end of this chapter to accelerate recovery time.

STEP B: HACK YOUR HEALTH (LAB TESTING)

If your assessment revealed "possible deficiency" or "support required," you likely have a weakened immune system and it's time to do more in-depth lab testing. This will provide you with valuable data that will establish a baseline for your current state of health and enable you to track your progress.

White Blood Cell (WBC) + Differential

The measurement of WBC + differential count evaluates two components: the total number of WBC present in your blood and the percentage of each type of WBC. WBC counts increase in response to infection, inflammation and possible trauma or stress. WBC counts decrease during chronic infections, dietary deficiencies, intense training, long-term stress or autoimmune diseases.

Secretory IgA (Stool)

A stool test assesses your intestinal levels of secretory IgA and determines the state of your first line of immune defence. This test can be done as a stand-alone test or as part of the Complete Stool Analysis (CSA). Deficiencies in sIgA levels are associated with increased risk of infection, increased risk of gut wall damage and yeast overgrowth. If test results reveal elevated levels of sIgA, they may reflect acute infection, food allergies and leaky gut, autoimmunity, parasitic infection, or increased exposure to environmental allergens.

Vitamin D

Vitamin D is essential for maintaining robust immunity over the winter months, as well as keeping your mood and cognitive function on track. If your vitamin D levels are low, you may get sick frequently, feel tired at the office or lack your normal energy and enthusiasm. Low levels of vitamin D are commonly found through the winter months in countries with long, dark winters. The normal range for vitamin D (25-hydroxy vitamin D) is between 75-250 nmol/L. The Vitamin D Council recommends your levels should be between 100-150nmol/L, which is difficult to maintain throughout the winter months without supplementation.

Food Allergies (IgG)

If you suspect food allergies (IgG) or note high sIgA levels on your stool test then getting tested for food allergies is important to identify the causes. There are two ways you can test IgG reactions: a blood test or the *Elimination Diet*.

IgG Food Sensitivity Testing

A pinprick blood test is compared with approximately 100 irritating foods and assessed for the presence of IgG antibodies. If your levels are elevated for a certain food, it indicates the presence of an adverse immune reaction. It is important to note that clients need to be consuming all the possible allergic foods before getting tested.

The Elimination Diet

The Elimination Diet requires you to eliminate all potential allergenic foods for two weeks. These foods include wheat, gluten, dairy, corn, eggs, soy, the nightshade family (tomatoes, white potatoes, eggplants, etc), and sugar. After eliminating these foods completely for 14 days, you begin to re-introduce the foods one at a time at every meal of the day for several days.

Reintroduce one specific food each day, paying close attention to any adverse symptoms you experience. A little detective work will allow you to identify any foods that may cause you problems. After you have identified the foods, eliminate them for 12-24 weeks, depending on the severity of the reaction.

STEP C: IMMUNITY SOLUTIONS

In order to build a robust immune system, you must provide the appropriate amount of support needed based on your *Immunity* self-assessment. Use the *Immunity Action Plan* table above, in Figure 5.7, to determine the appropriate levels required for you.

Level 1 Solution: Diet and Lifestyle

Diet

Food should always be your first-line therapy for correcting deficiencies in the body. A Modern Paleo diet provides abundant quantities of the most nutrient dense foods—meats, veggies, leafy greens, fruit, animal fats, etc.—to ensure you are meeting your daily requirements. The following is a list of immune building nutrients and the foods where they are commonly found.

Vitamin A

Cod liver oil is a rich natural source of vitamin A, along with many orange foods such as sweet potatoes, carrots, squash, cantaloupe and apricots. Be sure to include extra quantities when sick, rundown or through the winter months.

Vitamin C

Vitamin C significantly boosts immunity. It is vital for keeping tendons and ligaments strong and acts as a powerful antioxidant. Rich dietary sources of vitamin C include bell peppers, kale, parsley, broccoli, oranges and strawberries.

Zinc

Zinc is crucial in supporting the thymus gland and T-cell production. Be sure to include foods high in zinc in your diet, such as oysters, beef, lamb, crab, ginger, pumpkin seeds and dark chocolate. The food sources highest in zinc are animal proteins, which are plentiful in a Paleo diet.

Immunity Tea

Honey, ginger and cayenne are all heavyweight immune builders that can help fight off colds and flu. Honey is one of the strongest anti-bacterial agents found in nature and an excellent *demulcent*—a substance that coats a sore and dry throat—providing relief from cold and flu symptoms. Ginger and cayenne are considered "yang tonics" in Eastern medicine: pungent flavours that are warming to the body and stimulate circulation. Ginger plays a major role in preventing the adhesion of bacteria and viruses to your mucous membranes, preventing them from penetrating your immune defences.

A wonderful traditional immune recipe that can help you beat your next cold or flu is a mix of 1 tbsp of unpasteurized natural honey, with 1 tbsp of fresh grated ginger, and 1 tsp of lemon juice in one cup of boiling water. Stir and let simmer for three to five minutes. Sprinkle on some cayenne pepper to finish. This potent immune boosting decoction will get you back in the gym or the boardroom in no time.

Lifestyle

Optimal Hydration
While few scientific studies link dehydration directly to poor immunity, there is clear evidence that it reduces secretory IgA levels, your body's first-line of immune defence. Therefore, it is best practice to ensure optimal hydration to maintain optimal sIgA levels and robust immune defence.

Regularly performing a urinalysis test is a valuable tool for assessing your degree of hydration. Specific gravity measurements of 1.020 (+4) or greater reflect inadequate hydration. You should aim for 1.015 (+3) or below. To accomplish this, try consuming at least two litres of pure water daily, as well as plenty of water an hour or two before training (approximately two to four cups). A Paleo diet is loaded with fruit and vegetables, which contribute to keeping you properly hydrated.

Get Your Sleep
Sleep is critical for healthy immune function. You may notice the next time you feel rundown that you are tired early in the evening. Getting extra sleep when rundown or sick goes a long way to supporting your body and getting you back to health more quickly. Aim for at least eight hours of sleep per night, and do not be surprised if you need ten hours of sleep for several nights (if you are sick) before you get back to full health.

Reduce Stress

In England, the *British Journal of Sports Medicine* found that people under stress are twice as likely to get sick.[27] Busy workdays and intense training quickly increases cortisol stress levels, which takes a serious toll on your immunity. Meditation, yoga and breathing exercises are all wonderful tools for reducing cortisol levels and supporting more robust immunity.

PREVENTATIVE SUPPORT: ASTRAGALUS

If you are looking to do a little more to keep your immune system strong, try adding immune support from herbal medicines. One herb in particular—astragalus— is highly effective for this purpose.

Native to Northern China and Mongolia, astragalus has been used in Traditional Chinese Medicine (TCM) for centuries as a general tonic and to strengthen the body against disease. It supports the immune system and protects against colds and flu by helping to activate B-cells, T-cells, and natural killer cells of the adaptive immune system, increasing your resistance to viral infections.[28]

An added bonus is that astragalus shows great potential in anti-aging. A recent study showed that a certain chemical (TA-65) purified from astragalus has been shown to lengthen telomeres, which extend the lifespan of your DNA.[29] As you age, your telomeres shorten, adding wear and tear to your cells and accelerating aging. The ability to lengthen telomeres effectively extends the lifespan of your cells. My choice is the Astragalus Complex by Mediherb, which contains immune-boosting echinacea.

Level 2 Solution: Supplementation and Medicinal Mushrooms

Nutrient Supplementation

Vitamin D — 5,000-10,000 IU daily *(Get your levels re-tested after 12 weeks)*

Vitamin C — 1,000mg; 2-3 times daily

Zinc — 30mg; 2-3 times daily

Vitamin A — 10,000 IU daily

Glutamine — 10g post-training or bedtime

Medicinal Mushrooms

A combination of mushroom extract is a potent weapon against exercise-induced or work stress-induced immune depression. Mushrooms have been used for many centuries in TCM to battle colds and flu and support a healthy immune system. They contain a compound called beta-d-glucan (a polysaccharide), which exerts potent immune-enhancing effects.

Studies show that maitake stimulates natural killer (NK) cell activity, boosting both your innate first line of defence and adaptive seek-and-destroy immune responses to help fight off infections.[30] Their immune enhancing benefits are used extensively in cancer patients undergoing chemotherapy.

A combination of maitake, resihi, and shitake mushrooms should be used during your most intense training phase or at work when you feel as though you may be catching a cold or flu. If you get sick at the wrong time at work or during training, it will derail your success. Remember, only mushroom formulas using *"hot-water extracts"* should be used, as this form has the highest bioavailability and is proven to exert immune modulating effects.[31] My favourite choices are the *M/R/S Mushroom Formula* by Pure or the *Immune Formula* by JHS Naturals. Take two capsules, two or three times daily.

Level 3 Solution: Colostrum

Colostrum is a nutritional powerhouse and potent immune booster, containing 100 times more IgA and IgG immunoglobulins than cow's milk. Immunoglobulins are powerful immune factors that protect the mucosal linings of the gut and sinuses, helping to fight off foreign invaders.

Colostrum is a potent anti-bacterial, anti-viral and anti-fungal agent in your gut, helping to fight off colds and flu. A recent study in the *British Journal of Nutrition* examined the effects of colostrum supplementation on 20 male cyclists. Researchers wanted to find out whether or not the addition of colostrum could help prevent colds and flu, often experienced by endurance athletes when training at high intensity. The results showed that colostrum supplementation speeded up recovery and prevented decreases in innate immunity.[32] If your immune system is heavily taxed or you are peaking for a competition, add colostrum to your protocol. It's important to use only high-quality colostrum formulas to ensure optimal purity, my choice being *Teglecolostrum* by Douglas Labs. Take two to five grams daily.

IF ALLERGIES ARE PRESENT ADD QUERCETIN

Quercetin is part of the flavonoid family of compounds called flavonols, which are found naturally in vegetables and fruit. The average daily quercetin intake in a Western-type diet is approximately 14mg per day.[33] Quercetin inhibits food allergy responses by inhibiting the IgE immune reactions from mast cells and IgG immune reaction histamine release.

The most abundant food sources are apples, berries, onions, brassica family vegetables, grapes and tea. It also appears in significant quantities in the medicinal herb gingko biloba.[34] Quercetin supports healthy immune response via its potent antioxidant function, ability to regenerate glutathione and its anti-inflammatory capacity. If you need more robust support, supplement with 500mg two to three times daily during bouts of allergy.

ACUTE IMMUNITY PROTOCOL

Berberine is found naturally in a variety of plants, including the medicinal herb goldenseal. Goldenseal is classified as king of the mucous membranes in herbal medical texts for its exceptional anti-microbial activity, helping to fight off bacteria, viruses and parasites.[35] Best of all, it is able to exert these effects without harming good gut bacteria.

Adding this herb to your supplement regime when you are sick reduces the severity and duration of your cold or flu. Berberine helps to support healthy blood sugar, insulin and cholesterol levels. My choice for immunity is *Berbemycin* by Xymogen. The recommended dosage is 200mg, two or three times daily until symptoms resolve. Note: Berberine is very drying to the gut, so be sure to drink plenty of water to avoid constipation.

CASE STUDY—IMMUNITY

Anika, a 38-year-old marketing director, was referred to me several years ago with complaints that she was frequently sick during the winter months. This made it very difficult for her to keep up with the demands of her job. After a month-long flu, she finally decided to do something about it.

Anika's health history reveals that she struggles to fall asleep and averages only six hours of sleep per night. She typically works 60-70 hours per week, drinks three or four cups of coffee daily and frequently skips meals due to work. She travels twice a year to compete in marathons around the world, takes NSAIDs three or four times per week after her training and has experienced bouts of irritable bowel over the last ten years. She reports having had bad colds at least once a year that require a course of antibiotics. Figure 5.8 shows Anika's lab test results.

Lab Test	Normal Range	Anika's Levels	Significance
White Blood Cells (WBC)	4.0-11.00	3.8	Depressed immune function
Neutrophils	2.0-7.5	1.6	Low innate immunity
Vitamin D	75-250	45	Low vitamin D
Cortisol	170-720	150	Low morning cortisol
Secretory IgA (sIgA)	50-200	376	High – likely leaky gut & food allergies

Figure 5.8. Summary of Anika's Lab Test Results

Like most people, the cause of Anika's poor immunity was multi-factorial. Deficiencies and imbalances on multiple fronts led to her depleted immune army. First, I focused my attention on her digestive system, as 70% of the immune system is located there. The years of taking NSAIDs and antibiotics had destroyed Anika's gut flora and damaged the lining of her digestive tract, leading to a leaky gut. This condition heavily taxes the immune system, resulting in her elevated sIgA levels (376).

We removed the simple sugars and gluten from her diet for eight weeks, boosted her protein intake by adding eggs (at least three) or a protein shake for breakfast, and increased her consumption of healthy saturated fats such as coconut oil and ghee that act as anti-microbials to clean up the gut. I had Anika supplement with probiotics twice daily for eight weeks to re-establish healthy gut flora.

Next, Anika's hectic work and exercise schedule, combined with her lack of sleep, was the perfect recipe for over-training and exhaustion. We reduced her coffee intake to one daily (green tea to replace the other cups) and made sure she got to bed no later than midnight. Finally, we added medicinal mushrooms and vitamin D supplements to support a more robust innate immunity.

After the first week, Anika noticed her energy levels improve dramatically. She felt less sluggish upon rising, her motivation to workout returned and her month-long cold completely resolved. She made it through the rest of the winter months without catching any more colds or flu and completed the London marathon in a personal best time!

CHAPTER 6

INFLAMMATION—The Athlete's Enemy

In North America, the annual growth of chronic disease is on the rise with cancer (10 million), diabetes (14 million), autoimmune diseases (24 million), allergies (50 million), and cardiovascular disease (60 million) at the head of the pack. Exciting new research is uncovering the fact that inflammation may be the *root cause* of almost all chronic diseases.

It seems the hotter your internal inflammatory fire is burning, the more likely you are to suffer from poor health, weight gain and subpar performance. The troubling part is most people are completely unaware that the flames of inflammation are building-up inside them and leading them down the path to poor health, weight gain, and chronic disease.

Expert researchers now agree that if you can cool inflammation, you can dramatically improve your brain and cognitive function, fight off degenerative diseases, and upgrade your capacity to recover from exercise. In clinical practice, I often see the triad of chronic inflammation, digestive and immune dysfunction as the root cause for many client complaints. These systems are intricately linked and any dysfunctions will compromise your goal to achieve better health, a better body, or your performance potential.

How do you know if you suffer from too much inflammation? If you are overweight or carrying extra body fat around your mid-section, the fires of inflammation will burn hotter. If you suffer from dysbiosis or leaky gut, the fires of inflammation will burn hotter. If you have poor immunity, food allergies, or an autoimmune condition, the fires of inflammation will burn hotter.

On the other hand, you may have no overt symptoms that systemic inflammation is building-up inside you because it can be a silent condition.

What causes this destructive inflammation? The causes of inflammation are diverse. Inflammation can occur due to poor food choices (excessive sugars, carbs and processed foods), medications, poor digestion, chronic infections, high stress levels, nutrient deficiencies or overexposure to environmental toxins. This is an extensive list of potential causes for accelerating inflammation.

If you are striving to upgrade your health, improve body composition or increase performance, your goal should be to mitigate excessive and chronic inflammation. I will review the role of inflammation in the body and then discuss solutions for inflammation and how you can keep it at bay.

I. BACK TO BASICS—INFLAMMATION 101

The title of this chapter is a little misleading. The athlete's enemy is actually *not* inflammation but rather *chronic* inflammation. In truth, inflammation is a necessary and important reaction by your body to injury or infection, the general alarm bell that signals your immune system to take action. The classic signs of an inflammatory reaction are heat, redness, swelling, and pain—all of which are your body's best effort to resolve your injury or infection.

Chronic inflammation is a different story. Today, expert doctors and researchers believe that inflammation is the underlying cause of almost all chronic diseases. This is a very important finding.

Cytokines and Inflammation

Your inflammatory response is your body's first reaction when something goes wrong in the body. The characteristic fever, redness, malaise and pain is triggered by a group of immune system modulators called *cytokines* that exert powerful pro- and anti-inflammatory effects on your body.

Specific pro-inflammatory cytokines are responsible for kicking off the inflammatory reaction. The three principal cytokines are called *tumour necrosis factor alpha (TNF)*, *interleukin 1 (IL-1)* and *interleukin 6 (IL-6)*. How do they work? After injury, infection or an intense training bout, your innate immune system is activated, triggering an inflammatory response and the production of various cytokines. *Interleukin-1 (IL-1)* is a group of 11 different cytokines that are responsible for your inflammatory response to infection. They are produced in large quantities by the macrophages and monocytes of your immune system.

Interleukin-6 (IL-6) acts as *both* a pro- or anti-inflammatory cytokine, significantly increasing after damage to tissue (i.e., training or injury) or burns. It kicks off the production of pro-inflammatory prostaglandins (PGE2) and is a key immune communication cell that stimulates the production of other pro-inflammatory chemicals, most notably C-reactive protein (CRP), the most commonly used diagnostic lab marker for inflammation.

Finally, *tumour necrosis factor alpha* (TNF-a) is produced chiefly by macrophages and plays a key role in systemic inflammation. It is important in killing off cancer cells by inducing apoptosis (literally programming abnormal cells to terminate themselves), thereby limiting the spread of tumours, as well as being an important player in chronic inflammation.

Chronic Disease and Inflammation

In 2011, the prestigious *New England Journal of Medicine* published a review of the growing connection between chronic inflammation and the development of today's most common chronic diseases.[1] Close to one million people were analysed in the study that shed light on the link between elevated blood sugar, inflammation and the progression of degenerative chronic disease.

Almost every chronic disease—heart disease, obesity, diabetes, cancer and high blood pressure—has at its root a silent inflammatory process that accumulates over the years and accelerates the disease process. Regardless of whether you have high blood pressure, elevated cholesterol levels, cancer or diabetes, all diseases improve when inflammation is cooled. Therefore, cooling inflammation should be a top priority for all clients.

Inflammation and Weight Loss

In terms of weight loss, the current medical literature tells us that if you are overweight or obese, you have low-grade *systemic* inflammation. This constant internal fire disrupts your body's normal homeostasis, causing many of the adverse hormonal reactions that occur with weight gain.[2] The inflammation caused by weight gain starts the downward spiral that can make it much more difficult for you to shed those unwanted pounds and get your health back on track.

Inflammation and Athletes

Even if you are fit and healthy, you may not be exempt from the detrimental impacts of chronic inflammation. While a certain amount of exercise is fantastic for reducing inflammation, training intensely or preparing for a competition will quickly increase your inflammatory levels above the therapeutic threshold.

For athletes, controlling inflammation is critical to recovering from exercise because excessive muscular damage is detrimental to performance and recovery. It is also crucial for preventing nagging injuries from spiralling out of control and into more serious injuries that could hinder your ability to train and compete.

Whether you are striving to achieve a better body, a personal best race time or improve your overall health, controlling inflammation is a critical component of the *Paleo Project* paradigm.

II. HOW THINGS GO WRONG—CHRONIC INFLAMMATION

1. Weight Gain

2. Gluten

3. Painkillers (NSAIDs)

4. Digestion and Immune Dysfunction

5. Overtraining

The five most common factors seen in clinical practice that contribute to systemic inflammation are weight gain, gluten consumption, chronic use of NSAIDs (non-steroidal anti-inflammatory drugs), digestive or immune disturbances and over-training.

1) Weight Gain and Inflammation

Scientists used to think that fat was merely extra tissue just hanging around the body, taking up space and making our jeans fit more tightly. We no longer believe this. Fat is not inert. We now know that fat mass is actually a *biologically active* tissue.

What does this mean? Fat mass plays an *active role* in controlling important hormonal production in your body. The more body fat you are carrying, the greater the hormonal and inflammatory effects. New research shows that fat tissue functions like an endocrine organ, producing powerful hormones that exert a tremendous effect on your metabolism, inflammation and likelihood of chronic disease.[3]

Fat cells stimulate the production of a hormone called *leptin*, which is pro-inflammatory in nature.[4] Leptin talks to your brain in order to control your hunger. The more body fat you are carrying, the more leptin you will produce. This is your body's natural feedback mechanism designed to curtail your appetite.

Unfortunately, our modern diets have short-circuited this evolutionary adaptation. In the long term, excessive leptin production eventually leads to leptin resistance, similar to insulin resistance, when your brain no longer responds normally to the leptin signal.[5] At this point, weight-gain problems start for many people. Your normal leptin satiety signal gets scrambled so your body doesn't receive the message from your brain that says, "I am full" and you continue to crave and eat processed and sugary foods. This vicious cycle is seen in Figure 6.1.

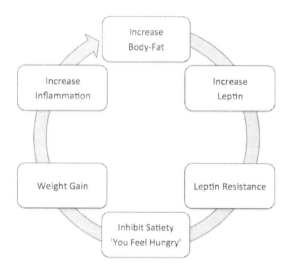

Figure 6.1. Leptin Resistance Cycle

Being overweight or obese leads to the reduction of another important hormone called *adiponectin*. This hormone improves the energy efficiency of your muscles, accelerating the rate your body can oxidize or "burn" fat for energy. The leaner you are, the more adiponectin you produce.[6] Therefore, the perfect storm for weight gain and inflammation is chronically high leptin and low adiponectin levels, making it much more difficult for you to lose weight and keep it off!

White Fat, Brown Fat and Inflammation

There are two types of fat in your body with dramatically different biological effects: white fat and brown fat.[7] What kind of fat are you made of?

White adipose tissue (WAT) is typically found around your mid-section and the accumulation of fat around your abdomen is considered the strongest risk factor for inflammation and chronic disease. If you have a beer belly or a muffin top, chances are your inflammation levels are high. The more white fat you are carrying, the greater your inflammatory levels.

In the lower body, it's a different story altogether. The excess accumulation of WAT in the lower body and around the hips (more typical in females), does not confer the same negative consequences for inflammation and disease.[8] This is why men with beer bellies have a far greater disease risk than women carrying extra weight around the hips.[5] It's not just the kind of fat you are made of but where your fat is located on your body that affects health and inflammation. Remember, WAT is very difficult to burn for energy, making it more difficult for you to lose weight.

In contrast, brown adipose tissue (BAT) can be more easily burned and used for energy. Whereas white adipose tissue contains one single large fat droplet, brown adipose tissue contains many small droplets and a high concentration of mitochondria.[6] These mitochondria are the fat-burning furnaces of your body, making BAT much more metabolically active tissue and giving it its characteristic brown colour. Brown fat has many more capillaries (tiny blood vessels) innervating it than white fat, making it much easier to burn for energy.

You can roughly determine your prevalence of BAT versus WAT by performing a skin fold caliper body-fat test (more on this in Chapter 9) or simply pinching your skin at your mid-section and hips. The thinner the pinch of skin is, the greater your levels of healthy BAT. The thicker the pinch, the greater are your levels of unhealthy WAT. In short, more brown fat and less white fat will make you healthier and accelerate your weight-loss progress.

New research suggests that the activation of BAT breakdown is mediated by your sympathetic fight or flight nervous system and the hormone leptin.[9] By supporting optimal function of these pathways you maximize your BAT to WAT ratio. This ratio is critically important if you want to achieve better body composition.

Athletes are not immune to this problem. If you compete in certain sports or higher weight classes such as football linemen, shot-putters, rugby players, Olympic weightlifters or any athlete who must maintain a higher fat mass to perform in his sport, you should be evaluating your BAT to WAT ratio in order to promote superior health, performance and recovery. In such cases, providing added anti-inflammatory support to help cool the increased pro-inflammatory pathways that occur as a result of increased weight and fat mass is highly recommended.

In summary, greater abdominal and visceral fat leads to increased levels of inflammation. At the end of this chapter, I outline solutions to cool this excessive inflammatory response.

2) Gluten and Inflammation

In recent years, the Paleo diet trend has been gaining significant momentum. The Modern Paleo Diet should be the foundation from which to improve your nutrition. It provides many profound health benefits: optimal protein intake, ideal omega-3 to 6 essential fat ratio, rich in vitamins and minerals (high nutrient density), plentiful source of fibre and loaded with electrolytes. In essence, the Paleo diet most closely resembles a diet in line with how we evolved. However, there is another major driving force behind the overwhelming success of an ancestral or Paleo approach to eating.

What's the secret? *The Paleo diet is a powerful tool for reducing inflammation.*

Quick history lesson. The consumption of grains began approximately 10,000 years ago, when humans began the agricultural revolution by harvesting grains to sustain larger groups of people living in villages. This meant that dietary staples shifted from primarily essential fats and proteins to one based on complex carbohydrates, such as wheat, rye and barley. These grains all contain the protein *gliadin*, one of two major proteins found in gluten.

New research is showing that the consumption of gluten may be problematic for weight loss, athletic performance and your overall health! In Chapter 4, we discussed the importance of optimal digestion and the detrimental effects of a leaky gut on your health and performance. The latest medical research shows that consuming foods that contain gluten may interfere with the function of an intestinal protein called *zonulin* and trigger leaky gut syndrome.

Zonulin is responsible for regulating your intestinal permeability by keeping your gut cells tightly packed. It essentially functions as the gatekeeper of your intestinal tract. The gliadin protein in gluten interferes with your zonulin function, leading to increased intestinal hyperpermeability or leaky gut.[10] It was once thought this occurred only in celiac patients (those with severe gluten intolerance), but new studies have revealed that it may be damaging to non-celiac populations (the rest of us) as well.

Let me explain this relationship in a little more detail. Your gut cells are held together by *tight junctions* that are constantly changing shape in order to absorb nutrients (paracellular absorption seen in Figure 6.2) and ensure that no pathogens or undigested proteins get through your gut wall and into the bloodstream. Zonulin's job is to tag the incoming molecules, labelling them as friendly so your immune system allows them free passage into the bloodstream, or tagging them as unfriendly or foreign invaders to be destroyed by your immune system.

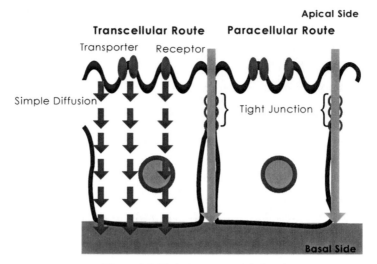

Figure 6.2. Tight Junctions and Zonulin

What does this have to do with gluten? The consumption of gluten directly interferes with zonulin function. When gluten attaches itself to the transport molecule CXCR3, it results in the release of zonulin, thus dissolving the *tight junctions* between your intestinal cells.[11] This opens up the floodgate to bacteria, viruses, toxins, undigested proteins and other pathogens to make their way into your bloodstream and trigger a major immune and inflammatory response by your immune response.

Weight Gain, Zonulin and Inflammation

Being overweight and obese affects your zonulin function. In a recent study, 173 men were assessed for their circulating zonulin levels, metabolic and inflammatory parameters. The results showed that overweight subjects (measured as increased BMI) and those with elevated waist-to-hip ratio had a significantly worse zonulin function.[12] Therefore, if you are carrying too much weight your digestion will suffer and so will your inflammatory levels.

This inflammatory connection was seen in subjects with poor zonulin function who also had elevations in lab markers fasting insulin, triglycerides, uric acid and IL-6, all of which are associated with chronic inflammation.

To summarize, if you are overweight or obese there is a strong likelihood that you have zonulin dysfunction, which translates into increased chances of a leaky gut and a greater risk of chronic inflammation. It's a horrible domino effect that reduces weight loss and contributes to poor health.

3) Painkillers and Inflammation

Non-steroidal anti-inflammatory drugs (NSAIDs) are the most common over-the-counter medication used to treat pain and inflammation. If you have pain from sitting at your desk all day, years of playing sports or a recent injury, chances are you are using NSAIDs to help cope with the pain. These injuries result in inflammation and pain syndromes that are persistent and interfere with your productivity and focus at work or in your favourite sport or activity. However, the NSAID solution that most people rely on comes with some serious consequences.

In 2012, a study from the Netherlands indicated the serious side effects of habitual NSAID users. Researchers found that people who regularly consumed NSAIDs had a high degree of intestinal tissue damage and significantly increased gut permeability or leaky gut.[13] The study revealed that the more NSAIDs you take, the greater your likelihood of developing a leaky gut. If over-the-counter painkillers are your go-to for treating pain, you are destroying your digestive system, the foundation of the *Paleo Project Pyramid,* and triggering a host of new problems.

A leaky gut is a performance killer that can lead to digestive distress, systemic inflammation and chronic over-activation of your immune system. This condition is often associated with joint pain, poor performance and slow recovery. Therefore, you should avoid taking NSAIDs unless it's absolutely necessary otherwise it's one step forward and three steps back. You are trading a minor problem today for major problems further down the road. The evidence from the Netherlands study was so compelling that researchers recommended discouraging the use of NSAIDs based on the scientific literature. Enough said.

NSAIDs and Ulcers

The excessive use of painkiller drugs wreaks havoc on your stomach, damaging the lining of the stomach wall and leading to the increased likelihood of stomach ulcers.[14] Ulcers are erosions of previously healthy tissue and the body's last-ditch attempt to expel toxins from the area. They are also extremely painful, so it's best to prevent them from occurring. Remember, protein digestion takes place primarily in your stomach, so even if you don't get an ulcer, damaging your stomach wall will compromise your digestion and ultimately your health, performance and recovery.

NSAIDs and Soft Tissue

Finally, another reason why NSAIDs are a poor choice is that they block the formation of new cartilage and soft tissue.[13] Most people take these drugs to help them heal after injury but don't realize that NSAIDs ultimately *inhibit* connective tissue formation in the long term—leaving you more susceptible to injury! Sounds crazy doesn't it, but unfortunately it's true.

Ironically, NSAIDs are the current treatment of choice for most professional sports team and endurance athletes. Intense training can trigger excessive inflammation and muscular damage, which translates into a greater degree of joint pain and muscle stiffness. Most people opt for the quick fix. They pop a painkiller (NSAID) and carry on with their day. Unfortunately, in life there is no such thing as a free lunch! There are many more negative long-term effects of relying on NSAIDs to curb your pain. The side effects are shown in Figure 6.3.

While NSAIDs are effective in the first five days or so after an injury during the inflammatory phase, after this point they can be detrimental to your joints and health. In spite of all of this clinical evidence, NSAIDs are typically the primary medication prescribed to relieve the pain of injuries and are commonly used for long-term care.

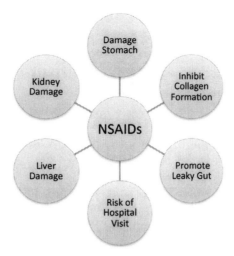

Figure 6.3. Side Effects of NSAID Use

4) Digestive and Immune Dysfunction

In the previous two chapters, I discussed the importance of digestion and immunity on your overall health and performance. Seventy
percent of your immune system is located in your gut; therefore, these
two systems are intricately linked to your inflammatory response. With
the increasing incidence of digestive disturbances, auto-immunity and
food allergies, it's imperative to ensure your digestion and immunity
are sound.

This is a major reason why digestion and immunity are at the base of
the *Paleo Project Pyramid*. If you work your way through the pyramid
step-by-step, you will maximize your chances of success. In short, if
your digestion or immunity is out of balance, you'll likely be stuck in
inflammation overdrive.

5) Overtraining

If you are training intensely, you need to pay special attention to controlling excessive inflammation. Although I described the therapeutic
nature of an inflammatory response, excessive muscular damage is
another common cause of chronic inflammation that can hamper your
recovery and therefore your future performance.

After a good training session or a long ride, you probably experience some muscular discomfort for a day or two. This mild muscular damage is called delayed onset muscle soreness (DOMS) and helps to trigger the growth of stronger muscle tissue. However, like most things in life, you can get too much of a good thing!

Excessive muscular damage from exercise that is too intense or too many hard training days in a row may cause excessive inflammation, which is not good for your muscles or your recovery. The key point to remember is that acute inflammation post-training does not peak until 24 hours after training, meaning after a hard workout today, you'll still be experiencing inflammation most of the next day and possibly during your subsequent workout.[15] Keep this in mind next time you decide to start a new exercise regime or plan on attacking an intense training phase. You'll reap major rewards if you add some of the anti-inflammatory solutions listed in the next section—it will go a long way to improving your recovery, personal best time or maximum lift.

III. THE PALEO PROJECT—INFLAMMATION PLAN

The best strategy for cooling excessive inflammation is to deal with the root causes. This means addressing the key factors contributing to your inflammation, which include weight gain, gluten consumption, painkillers (NSAIDs), digestive/immune dysfunction and overtraining. Other common factors include poor dietary choices (refined sugars, excess carbs and bad fats), lack of exercise, high stress, chronic infections, poor gut health, environmental allergies and toxins.

STEP A: SELF-ASSESSMENT

Complete the *Inflammation* self-assessment and incorporate the corresponding *Inflammation Action Plan* appropriate for you in Figure 6.4.

Inflammation Self-Assessment

- Is your life very busy or stressful?

- Do you have arthritis?

- Do you have dermatitis (eczema, acne, rashes)?

- Do you have IBS or ulcerative colitis?

- Do you have food, seasonal or environmental allergies?

- Are you overweight or have significant belly-fat?

- Do you drink more than three glasses of alcohol per week?

- Do you exercise LESS THAN 30 minutes three times per week?

- Do you have an autoimmune disease (rheumatoid arthritis, lupus, hypothyroidism)?

- Do you have diabetes, heart disease or have you ever had a heart attack?

STEP A: SELF-ASSESSMENT		STEP B: HACK YOUR HEALTH	STEP C: INFLAMMATION SOLUTIONS		
Grade	Score	Lab Testing	Level 1 (Diet + Lifestyle)	Level 2 (Curcumin + Fish Oils)	Level 3 (Resveratrol)
Pass	0-2	n/a	✔	n/a	n/a
Possible Deficiency	3-6	✔	✔	✔	n/a
Support Required	7+	✔	✔	✔	✔

Figure 6.4. Inflammation Action Plan

STEP B: HACK YOUR HEALTH (LAB TESTING)

Laboratory markers for inflammation serve as a valuable tool for assessing your degree of inflammation. These simple blood tests take the guesswork out of wondering whether your current diet, exercise and supplement protocol is working for you.

CRP (Blood)

One of the primary markers of systemic inflammation is called *C-reactive protein* (CRP). As your body fat increases, so do your CRP levels. A recent study by the *Harvard Medical School* showed a strong relationship between consuming high-glycemic carbs (white bread, cereal, baked goods) and elevated CRP levels.[16] Eating too many carbs, especially the refined and processed kind, quickly leads to weight gain and subsequent inflammation. By avoiding or limiting processed and sugary foods that spike blood sugar and insulin levels, you will start to shift the inflammatory response.

The latest medical studies show that as you grow older your levels of inflammatory markers tend to increase and elevations in CRP are associated with a 300% increase risk of death.[17] The more inflamed you are, the harder your body has to work to maintain overall health and recovery. Ideal levels of CRP are less than 0.8.

If you are training intensely or performing CrossFit style training, then specific lab markers for muscular inflammation such as lactate dehydrogenase (LDH) and creatine kinase (CK) should be tested regularly to avoid overtraining.

Uric Acid (Blood)

Uric acid is a pro-inflammatory molecule produced in the body as a by-product of purine metabolism, a group of compounds that build your DNA. High levels are associated with chronic inflammation and increased risk of gout and kidney stones. Normal levels of uric acid are less than 0.35 mmol/L or 5.0mg/dL.

Homocysteine (Blood)

Homocysteine is a protein that has been shown to increase in those with elevated inflammatory levels and insulin dysfunction. High levels are associated with increased risk of heart disease, stroke and Alzheimer's disease. The optimal value is less than 6.3.

STEP C: INFLAMMATION SOLUTIONS

Use the *Inflammation Action Plan* table in Figure 6.4 to determine the recommended levels of support for you. Remember, you need to *control* inflammation, not eliminate it entirely.

Level 1 Solution: Diet and Lifestyle

Improve Leptin Sensitivity

If leptin resistance takes root, you will gain more weight and subsequently increase your inflammatory levels. This hormonal imbalance can easily become a vicious weight-gain cycle. How can you reverse the process? Improving your blood sugar and insulin balance is the first step (more on this in Chapter 7—Insulin). Next, aim to get the right amount of sleep every night, 7 to 8.5 hours, as this is shown to significantly improve your leptin sensitivity.[6]

Increase Adiponectin Levels

Improving your diet is an excellent way to kick-up your fat-burning adiponectin levels. Try including more dietary monounsaturated fats such as extra-virgin olive oil and avocados to help boost your levels (yes, that's right, eating fat will make you slimmer!).

Starting an exercise regime or increasing your activity levels is another proven strategy to increase adiponectin. Whether it's walking to work, taking the stairs instead of the elevator or jumping into a new training routine, movement is crucial for increasing adiponectin and helping to cool inflammation.

Eliminate Gluten

Eliminating gluten from your diet is a great way to reduce inflammation. Start by replacing breads and pastas with cruciferous vegetables and leafy greens. Pound for pound these vegetables are much more nutrient dense than breads and wheat-containing grains, meaning you get a lot more vitamin, mineral and nutrient bang for your buck than you would in breads.

Next, try substituting more root vegetables like sweet potatoes, yams, yucca (cassava), white potatoes, parsnips, beets and carrots for breads and pastas. Short-grain brown rice is a great choice because it's loaded with nutrients and keeps the gut healthy. The Modern Paleo diet is the perfect platform for cooling inflammation. (Remember, it's all about moderation. If your diet is laden with breads and pastas, start by gradually reducing your intake. Try one or two days without these foods and when you feel ready, increase the number of gluten-free days in your week.)

Eat More Fish

The extra-long-chain fatty acids (EPA/DHA) found in fish exert powerful anti-inflammatory effects through the production of hormone-like chemicals called prostaglandins.[18, 19] The fish highest in omega-3 fats are black cod, salmon, mackerel, anchovies, sardines and herring. A serving of fish typically contains approximately 750-1000mg EPA/DHA.

Of course, it is not enough just to increase your omega-3 intake. You must also reduce your omega-6 intake (nuts, vegetable oils, processed foods) in order to achieve the optimal ratio of omega-6 to omega-3 fats (3:1 to 1:1). By limiting your omega-6 intake— via reducing processed foods and omega-6 rich oils discussed in Chapter 2, you will reduce the pro-inflammatory nature of these fats. Once again, adopting a Modern Paleo diet or adding more Paleo-based meals to your regime will naturally restore this common imbalance.

Drink More Green Tea

Green tea is a natural source of over fifty anti-inflammatory compounds and has been shown to mitigate post-exercise muscular inflammation.[20] It's a great alternative to coffee, so try taking one or two days a week off coffee and adding green tea to your regimen. If you drink more than one cup of coffee per day, going cold turkey may be too much for you. If this is the case, try substituting green tea for your last cup of coffee.

Green tea is a potent antioxidant and terrific source of the amino acid *l-theanine*, which helps to relax the nervous system. This is extremely important for people working busy, strenuous jobs and anyone training frequently in the week. Aim to drink one to three cups of green tea per day and spread them out throughout the day for continuous anti-inflammatory support (nothing after 5 p.m.).

Balance Gut Flora

Eat foods that help to promote the growth of good probiotic bacteria in your gut. As I discussed in Chapter 4, dysbiosis and leaky gut are sure-fire ways to spread inflammation in the body. In order to maintain a healthy gut, include more *fermented* foods in your diet. For example, plain yogurt (avoid the sweetened stuff), kefir, sauerkraut, kimchee, natto miso, tamari sauce and kombucha tea are all great options to maintain a well-balanced gut.

Eat More Anti-Inflammatory Herbs

Ginger packs a powerful anti-inflammatory punch. It is a natural COX-2 inhibitor just like ibuprofen or naproxen, but it does not damage your gut.[21, 22] It's a great addition to your diet to help cool inflammation and it provides the added benefit of supporting superior digestion and immunity. For this reason, ginger is one of my favourite herbs for supercharging the body and keeping all your systems—digestive, immune, inflammatory—running smoothly. New research has shown that ginger, along with turmeric and rosemary, greatly reduce inflammatory markers after only seven days of consumption.[23] Include daily as a tea, use it when juicing or add it to your cooking.

Hot peppers can do more for you than just spice up your chili! *Capsaicins* are members of the nightshade family of plants and have special anti-inflammatory properties. They do not function like COX-2 inhibiting NSAID drugs. Instead, they interact with a receptor in the brain called TRPV (transient-receptor-potential vallinoid—now that is a mouthful!).[24] To reap the anti-inflammatory benefits, simply sprinkle cayenne on your meals, just like salt or black pepper. This will help cool inflammation and provide a nice metabolic boost.

Level 2 Solution: Fish Oils and Curcumin

Fish Oils

Supplementing with fish oils is a good idea if inflammation is a concern because it's difficult to achieve the therapeutic dose needed to cool your inflammation from food alone. Unless you are eating two pieces of cold, deep-water fatty fish daily, it's best to add an omega-3 supplement rich in EPA/DHA until your symptoms improve. You can do that by taking a daily dose of 1,500-3,000mg EPA/DHA.

Curcumin (Turmeric)

Curcumin is the active component in the powerful anti-inflammatory herb turmeric and should be a key part of everyone's anti-inflammatory arsenal. This amazing herb inhibits an array of inflammatory enzymes: COX-2, TxA2 and NF-KB. It is terrific for reducing high levels of muscular inflammation caused by intense training.[25]

Curcumin supports a healthy liver by keeping your detoxification pathways running smoothly. Finally, this wonderful anti-inflammatory herb does NOT exert the negative side effects commonly seen with painkiller drugs: leaky gut, ulcer formation and inhibition of soft tissue reformation. This is a major bonus! Take 800mg per day.

Level 3 Solution: Resveratrol

Resveratrol is the active compound in red wine. It's one of the main reasons behind the French Paradox—the notion that the French have superior health despite their penchant for smoking and a high fat diet (although, by now you realize that high fat is good for you!). Resveratrol is responsible for many of red wine's beneficial health properties: improving neurological and cardiovascular function, boosting metabolism and fighting cancer. Resveratrol is found naturally in grapes, berries and peanuts.

Classified as a polyphenol, resveratrol has strong anti-inflammatory properties, inhibiting the COX-2 and LOX inflammatory pathways that make it a great choice for reducing joint pain.[26] A recent study of

20 professional male basketball players found that those supplementing with resveratrol had significant reductions in *pro-inflammatory* TNF and IL-6 compared to a placebo after six weeks.[27]

If weight loss is your goal, incorporating resveratrol in your regimen is highly beneficial because it not only reduces inflammation but also improves insulin sensitivity and post-meal blood glucose levels.[28] This means if you have a beer belly or muffin top, you will benefit greatly from adding resveratrol to your regimen. Not only that, but resveratrol has potential anti-aging properties, boosting energy metabolism and mitochondrial health via activation of the SIRT 1 pathway.[29] Looks as though the French are on the right track! Take 50-100mg per day.

CASE STUDY—INFLAMMATION

Scott, a 42-year-old executive, came to me wanting to lose weight and improve his performance in the gym. He was a type-A personality, very driven and successful but had struggled since turning 40 to maintain his lifestyle, desired body weight and gym performance.

Scott would entertain clients for dinner most nights of the week, he survived on less than six hours of sleep per night, trained five days a week, and struggled with intense sugar and salt cravings. He also had chronically sore joints and generally felt tired all the time. Highlights of his lab test results are shown in Figure 6.5.

Lab Test	Normal Range	Scott's Levels	Significance
CRP-hs	Less than 1.0	4.2	High - reflects high levels of systemic inflammation
Uric Acid	Less than 0.35	0.50	High - reflects high levels of systemic inflammation
Homocysteine	Less than 11.4	10	High Normal - sign of systemic inflammation
ALT	12-49	70	High liver enzymes - reflects heavily taxed liver
LDH	120-246	320	High - reflects high levels of inflammation & possible excessive muscular damage

Figure 6.5. Summary of Scott's Lab Test Results

Scott's body–fat percentage was relatively high for his activity level (18%) and unfortunately most of this was around his mid-section. The weight gain, intense training and high alcohol intake was leading to systemic inflammation. Scott was eight weeks away from his summer vacation and was ready to dive headfirst into any protocol that was going to improve things.

Over the next eight weeks, Scott cut out all the alcohol from his diet, cut back to one coffee per day, and dramatically increased his protein and healthy fats intake while eliminating simple sugars, bread and pasta. He added high dose curcumin, resveratrol and fish oil supplementation to combat inflammation and dampen his joint pain.

Luckily for Scott, he could afford a meal service to deliver all his food—three Paleo meals a day over the next eight weeks. His compliance was exceptional and so were his results. He lost 5% body fat, eliminated his intense cravings, slept better at night and best of all, his training numbers were going back up. His joints felt much better performing compound exercises such as squats and deadlifts, and his muscle soreness post-exercise was no longer debilitating.

Stronger and leaner than before, Scott achieved a personal best in the gym and felt great on his vacation. While he still enjoys red wine a few nights a week, he has now found the right balance to maintain progress.

CHAPTER 7

INSULIN—The Athlete's Builder

We are in the midst of a weight-gain epidemic. In the last 30 years, the obesity rate in North America has tripled and three-quarters of the population is now classified as overweight or obese. In Europe and Asia the numbers are trending in the same direction. It seems the overconsumption of carbohydrates and notably sugars from processed foods and drinks is wreaking havoc on our bodies. Incredibly, over 80% of processed foods have sugar added to them!

The World Health Organization (WHO) has stated that by the year 2050 one-third of the global population will develop type-II diabetes (the inability to effectively process dietary sugars). This is truly stunning. The trend is so alarming that scientists have coined the new term *diabesity* to describe how dysfunctions in blood sugar and insulin function rapidly lead to weight gain, obesity and ultimately type-II diabetes. This generation will be the first to live a shorter life span than their parents!

Today, new research highlights that insulin affects *how you think* and *how you feel*. The WHO predicts that by 2050, one-third of the world population will be categorized as clinically depressed. This parallel prediction of depression and diabetes rates is not a coincidence. Your brain and your blood sugars are intimately connected.

The WHO has issued recommendations to governments in Canada and the USA to reduce sugar consumption to less than 10% of your total caloric intake. Unfortunately, while the science clearly indicates we need to reduce our intake, processed food companies seem to wield more power than government regulators. The recommendations of expert researchers at the WHO were ultimately removed at the last minute by government.

Whether you are trying to lose weight, compete at a high level in your sport or improve your general health, it's important to understand how the blood sugar hormone insulin works because this will lay the framework for your success in the long term.

I. BACK TO BASICS—INSULIN 101

Insulin Sensitivity—Your Carbohydrate Efficiency

Insulin is an *anabolic* hormone; it tells your body to *build* tissue. It is produced by the pancreas and responsible for lowering your blood sugars by stimulating the uptake of carbohydrates into your cells. It does this by telling receptors located inside muscle and fat cells (called glucose transporters or GLUT) to come up to the cell surface to absorb the glucose molecules. The GLUT receptors are the lock and key mechanism that allows glucose to enter cells.

Every cell in your body needs glucose for energy. When your body is functioning optimally, this system is very efficient and you are referred to as *insulin sensitive*. This is typically seen in healthy and active people, well-trained athletes and those with a lower body-fat percentage.

If you are out of shape, overweight or obese, your insulin sensitivity tends to suffer. This means that your GLUT receptors are no longer as efficient at getting the glucose into your cells. Effectively, they become lazy. This inefficiency is called *insulin insensitivity* and forces your body to produce more insulin than it would normally have to—not a good recipe for improving your health or losing weight.

If this inefficiency becomes more severe, you may develop *insulin resistance*. A person who is insulin resistant requires even greater outputs of insulin to make up for their severe insulin insensitivity. The result is chronically elevated insulin levels. Unfortunately, this means more work for your pancreas (to produce insulin) to cope with constantly high blood sugar levels. This is not good for your waistline, performance or overall health!

Insulin and Fat-Burning

Insulin plays a key role in a cascade of biochemical reactions that control your ability to burn fat. Remember, insulin is a building hormone and when produced in abundance it will make you bigger and stronger (from training) or just fatter (from inactivity).

Let me explain. Hormone sensitive lipase (HSL) is your primary *fat-burning* hormone. The HSL enzyme needs to be turned on (like a light switch) by an enzyme called *cyclic adenosine monophosphate* (cAMP) for you to be in fat-burning mode. Elevated insulin and blood sugar levels lower cAMP levels, telling your body to turn OFF your fat-burning ability.[1]

This is one of the most common reasons why people struggle to lose weight. It's also a major reason why the typical high-carb breakfast (i.e., orange juice, cereal, muesli, etc.) is blocking your fat-burning potential. Breads and cereals turn into sugars in your body, just like candy or a can of soda, raising insulin levels and leaving you stuck in fat-building mode.

Excess insulin contributes to weight gain in another way, turning on *lipogenic* or *fat building* enzymes in your body. This further suppresses your body's ability to burn fat for energy. If you are inactive, sitting at a desk all day or eating a lot of processed foods, chronically high insulin levels will promote packing on extra pounds very quickly. All those extra calories from mid-afternoon sugary snacks and lattes will be directed to your belly and hips, which are your body's primary fat stores. Your energy levels and mood will suffer as you continue along the weight-gain spiral. Remember, the better your insulin control, the greater your chances of success in your quest for weight loss.

Symptoms of Insulin Excess

The first physical signs of insulin dysfunction and blood sugar irregularities are complaints of weakness, sluggishness and fatigue. You may feel the need to eat something sweet or crave a caffeinated drink to keep your energy levels up. Another common symptom is the inability to maintain focus and concentration, particularly at work. You may experience this as difficulty staying on task or bouts of irritability toward co-workers.

Physical symptoms can also been seen. If you experience *puffiness*, especially noticeable at the wrists and ankles, you may have elevated insulin levels, because high insulin leads to increased sodium retention and ultimately greater water retention. Water retention quickly increases the numbers on your scale.

Athletes and so-called skinny people are not exempt from possible insulin and blood sugar dysfunction. Intense training or many days exercising may leave you constantly craving simple sugars or processed carbohydrates through the day. You may be consuming more than you should.

Many people believe because they are active or already thin they can disregard this keynote symptom. Over time, this may also lead to poor insulin sensitivity and peaks and valleys in your blood-sugar levels. If you experience a noticeable *energy crash* after eating a high-carb meal, this is an early sign of insulin dysfunction. Other common symptoms are shown in Figure 7.1.

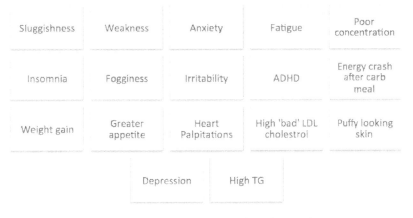

Sluggishness	Weakness	Anxiety	Fatigue	Poor concentration
Insomnia	Fogginess	Irritability	ADHD	Energy crash after carb meal
Weight gain	Greater appetite	Heart Palpitations	High 'bad' LDL cholestrol	Puffy looking skin
	Depression	High TG		

Figure 7.1. Common Symptoms of Insulin Dysfunction

The Benefits of Insulin

Insulin is not inherently bad. It's simply doing its job, which is signalling your body to go into *building* mode. Unfortunately, poor food choices and inactivity can leave you stuck in fat-building mode, rather than muscle-building mode!

Insulin exerts two powerful benefits:

- It's an *anabolic* hormone that stimulates lean muscle protein synthesis.

- It's powerfully *anti-catabolic*, preventing excessive muscle tissue breakdown after exercise.

If you can harness these tremendous benefits, you can transform your body, achieve better health and supercharge your performance in the gym or on the playing field. The key is all in the timing!

After a workout, you typically want to stimulate a rise of insulin by consuming liquid nutrition or food. Your muscles are primed to soak up a carbohydrate + protein shake or meal to replenish your muscle glycogen stores and increase the rate of amino acid absorption into muscle tissue.

How does exercise improve this response? Weight training and high-intensity interval training (HIIT) both trigger the release of glucose receptors (GLUT-4) normally dormant in your muscle cells.[2] These receptors are somewhat lazy and normally hang out in the interior of your cells. But weight training and HIIT exercise stimulate them to come up to the cell surface so your muscles can *soak up* the ingested carbohydrates. That's right—your muscle cells preferentially take up the carbs to restock glycogen stores. This incredible adaptation allows you to steer your carbohydrate consumption *toward* your muscles and *away* from your fat stores.

Insulin is powerfully *anti-catabolic*. When you exercise, your body must break down or catabolize tissue to produce fuel for energy while you train. Cortisol levels increase during exercise (which is a natural process) but should return to baseline soon after training. By increasing the *anabolic insulin* hormone after exercise, you can quickly decrease the *catabolic cortisol* hormone, preserving your precious muscle mass and improving recovery after training.

Problems start when your cortisol levels remain elevated post-training. This occurs due to high training intensity, high training volume or toward the end of an intense training phase. In the short term, you'll lose valuable muscle mass and glycogen stores. In the long term, elevated cortisol will tax your adrenal glands and lead to fatigue, poor recovery and disruption of deep sleep (more on this in Chapter 8—Cortisol).

Therefore, your primary goal immediately after exercise is to reduce this training-induced elevation in cortisol. Consuming a post-exercise carbohydrate + protein shake not only supports rebuilding lean muscle but also triggers a rise in insulin that quickly lowers high cortisol levels post-training.[3]

II. HOW THINGS GO WRONG—INSULIN DYSFUNCTION

Why are insulin dysfunction and the development of diabetes—the absolute endpoint of blood-sugar dysfunction—now so common-place? The truth is there are a number of reasons that contribute to this imbalance; however, it is widely believed by expert researchers in the field that obesity is the root cause behind blood sugar and insulin dysfunction and subsequently the development of type-II diabetes. In North America and Europe, it is thought to account for 70-90% of the patients with diabetes.[4]

The enormous increase in sugars added to processed foods has contributed tremendously to the epidemic of weight gain. However, it's not just your diet that is leading to insulin dysfunction—lifestyle factors such as stress and sleep also contribute to dysfunctions in blood sugars, insulin and ultimately weight gain.

The following is a list of the top five reasons for high blood sugars and insulin dysfunction:

1. Too Much HFCS

2. Too Many Carbs

3. Sugar Addiction

4. Lack of Sleep

5. Stress

1) Too Much High Fructose Corn Syrup (HFCS)

High fructose corn syrup (HFCS) is a synthetically produced sugar that is added to most juices, drinks and processed foods to increase sweetness. To make HFCS, corn undergoes an enzymatic process that converts the naturally occurring glucose into fructose, which significantly raises its level of sweetness. Why do companies do this? It's all about their bottom line. HFCS is a very cheap way to make processed snacks taste more palatable and in the 1980s when low-fat diets were all the rage, it was a crucial piece of the puzzle to make low-fat processed foods taste palatable. Table sugar (sucrose) is two or three times more expensive than HFCS, making HFCS the more attractive option for companies looking to improve their profits.

Unfortunately, the increasing consumption of HFCS interferes with leptin signalling—your body's satiety signal—thus contributing to expanding waistlines and increased body fat. How does this happen? Let me explain.

Table sugar or sucrose is a disaccharide made up of one fructose molecule linked to one glucose molecule. It's a 50:50 split. The major difference with HFCS is that it contains much more fructose, anywhere from a 60:40 split all the way up to 90% fructose to only 10% glucose. This ratio does not normally occur in nature.

Next, when you combine high fructose intake with excessive caloric intake, your liver acts as a sugar sponge. Fructose quickly fills up your liver glycogen stores and the overflow must be converted to a fat (palmitic acid), which then travels to your brain. As levels increase in the brain they scramble your body's normal leptin satiety cues, leading to *leptin resistance.* This results in uncontrolled eating, excessive caloric intake and weight gain.

Renowned pediatric endocrinologist Dr. Robert Lustig from the *University of California* shed new light on the damaging effects of high fructose consumption when his YouTube lecture *"Sugar: The Bitter Truth"* went viral in 2009. He explained that rats fed a high fructose diet (60% of their total daily calories) rapidly converted carbohydrates to fat via a process called *de novo lipogenesis (DNL).* As a result, they gained weight very quickly![5] He also found that when fructose was consumed in large quantities, it becomes incredibly toxic to the liver.

Therefore, if you are overweight or out of shape you *must* avoid high fructose corn syrup found in almost all processed foods and drinks—everything that comes in a box or can.

SHOULD I AVOID FRUIT IF I AM OVERWEIGHT?

If HFCS is bad, does this mean you should avoid fruit as well? The answer is all about the dose. For example, an apple contains approximately 10g of fructose compare to a can of soda pop that contains 25g. A banana contains about 7g of fructose compared to a whopping 62g from a large soda pop at a fast food chain!

Sugary drinks contain massive concentrations of fructose (HFCS); therefore, you should avoid them completely. In contrast, fruit contains naturally occurring fibre that slows the releases of sugars into the bloodstream. This does not cause the same problems as the artificial HFCS. Fruit also provides a wealth of vitamins, minerals and key nutrients that satiate the appetite and actually improve blood-sugar control.

HFCS AND DYSBIOSIS

New research is revealing another adverse effect of HFCS consumption— its ability to alter healthy gut microflora. The Institute of Food in Switzerland demonstrated strong connections between high fructose intake, altered gut bacteria and weight gain.[6] Researchers discovered HFCS changes the balance of beneficial gut bacteria and promotes the build-up of bad gut bacteria. This major shift causes intestinal dysbiosis—an imbalance of good to bad gut bacteria—and triggers a pro-inflammatory effect on your liver that promotes insulin resistance. These factors derail your health, weight loss and performance goals.

2) Too Many Carbs (Don't *Just* Blame Fructose)

Dr. John Sievenpiper, M.D. of *St. Michael's Hospital* at the *University of Toronto,* has been studying the effects of fructose intake in humans (not rats) and his work has shed new light on the "high fructose consumption equals fat gain" discussion.

First, Dr. Sievenpiper shows that the concentration of fructose fed to the rats in the original studies was astronomically high. Humans cannot consume 60% of their calories from fructose, like the rats in the experiment. Based on national survey studies, even the highest fructose consumers are only getting 20% of the total caloric intake from fructose (this is still very high, but nowhere near the 60% intake by the animals in the study), making it virtually impossible for most people to consume triple this amount![7]

Next, Dr. Sievenpiper's research found that when two groups consumed the same number of calories (iso-caloric diet), the group being fed a high fructose load (20% of total calories) experienced no significant weight changes when compared to the group consuming a high glucose load (20% of total calories).[7] Although too much HFCS is still bad, it seems that too much sugar is simply too much sugar, regardless of where it comes from!

The reality is that your body was never designed to cope with such massive intakes of carbohydrates and sugar. Unfortunately, the typical Western diet is already loaded with carbohydrates, particularly at breakfast time when cereals, toast, bagels, jam and orange juice are classic staples. *The average North American consumes a whopping 160 pounds of sugar every year!* Compare this to 100 years ago, shown in Figure 7.2, when the average intake was approximately 40 pounds, or one-quarter of today's intake. If you sit at a desk all day or are mainly sedentary, chronically high insulin levels lead to constant cravings for more carbs and ultimately weight gain.

Around the world, most people are unaware just how much their diet revolves around sugars and carbohydrates. Why so much emphasis on carbs? Carbohydrates exert the greatest impact on your insulin levels; therefore, the massive overconsumption of carbs and sugars adds fuel to the insulin dysfunction fire. In 1980, not a single 13-year-old was diagnosed with adult-onset diabetes (type-II diabetes). Today, there are over 50,000 13-year-old kids diagnosed with adult-onset diabetes, forcing doctors to stop using the term *adult-onset* because the disease is so commonplace in kids. Imagine, a disorder once thought only possible in adulthood is now commonplace in children!

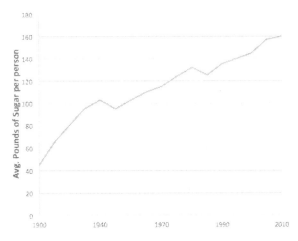

Figure 7.2. Average Sugar Consumption in the 1900s

The excess sugar doesn't just throw off your insulin control. It also inhibits your satiety hormone *leptin*. Studies confirm that high circulating leptin levels in overweight and obese individuals act similarly to chronically high insulin levels. You become resistant to the leptin signal and *leptin resistance* takes root. Leptin resistance is when your brain no longer receives the satiety signal. You keep craving more carbs and sugars, thus exacerbating the weight-gain cycle.

In 2012, an Australian study examined the effects of varying *macronutrient intake*—the ratio of carbs, proteins and fats—on hunger hormones in lean and obese individuals. In the lean group, they were most satiated and least hungry after the high-protein meal, high-fat meal compared to high-carbohydrate, low-protein meal.[8] They also consumed fewer calories and snacked less frequently. In the obese group, they consumed far more calories after high-carb meals and were most satiated and least hungry after the high-protein meals (fat intake was not as crucial as protein intake for blunting hunger in obese individuals).

TOO MANY ARTIFICIAL SWEETENERS

Sucralose is a sugar alcohol, a synthetic and chemically modified version of a sugar designed to taste sweet (200x sweeter than sugar) with little caloric impact. It is made in a laboratory when sugar is treated with three chlorine compounds (trityl chloride, acetic anhydride, hydrogen chlorine, thionyl chloride) and methanol in the presence of dimethylformamide, 4-methyl-morpholine, toluene, methyl isobutyl ketone, acetic acid, benzyltriethylammonium chloride and sodium methoxide. (Does that sound natural?)

Manufacturers prefer sucralose because it increases sweetness in products and has negligible caloric impact. People love "low-calorie" snacks, thinking they are best for weight loss. However, while it does not significantly impact your blood sugars, it does dramatically increase your insulin levels.[9] It's like a magic trick—remove the carbs and the calories and people will think it's a healthier option. Unfortunately, by elevating insulin levels, it directly inhibits your ability to burn fat.

Too much sucralose leads to loose stools, diarrhea and even anal leakage! Other common side effects include headaches, numbness, muscle ache and stomach pain. Doesn't sound like such a good option to me. Does it sound like it to you?

In 2012, a study showed that the breakdown of sucralose into the water table harms the motor function of crustaceans, which suggested a toxic or over-stimulatory activation that researchers believed should be considered as a warning against exposure.[10] This has led many to question the long-term safety of sucralose. The scientific community has advised that further testing is needed on sucralose and other sweeteners to ensure they are not detrimental to overall health.[11]

3) Sugar Addiction

If we know that sugar is not good for us, why do we still consume it? Why does an alcoholic continue to drink too much alcohol? The answer is simple—addiction. An overlooked factor contributing to the weight gain and obesity epidemic permeating the globe is sugar addiction.

While it's widely accepted that recreational drugs such as cocaine are extremely addictive and harmful to the brain and body, new research suggests the negative impact of sugar addiction could actually be WORSE than this notorious narcotic.[12] Would you believe that sugar is *more* addictive than cocaine? Most people are unaware of how powerfully addictive sugar can be—eight times more addictive than cocaine, shown in Figure 7.3—but new research has uncovered its powerful influence on your cravings and behaviour.

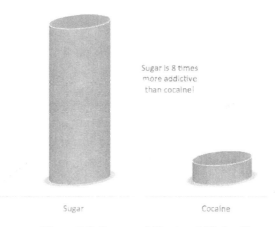

Sugar is 8 times more addictive than cocaine!

Sugar   Cocaine

Figure 7.3. Sugar and Cocaine Addiction Rate

Researchers in France tested this hypothesis in a recent study by comparing the addictive power of sugar versus that of cocaine. Incredibly, the authors found that the overwhelming majority of mice preferred the sweet sugar reward to the highly addictive cocaine reward. When researchers then decided to increase the cocaine dose to see if this would influence addiction, they were surprised to find that the mice still preferred the sugar!

Finally, they decided to make it even *more* difficult for the mice to obtain the sugar reward and easier for the cocaine reward. Would you believe the mice still preferred to struggle and work harder to obtain the sweet sugar reward rather than go for the much easier cocaine reward?

These results demonstrate that humans and animals are not well adapted to sweet-tasting foods with high concentrations of sugar. They identified specific sweet receptors called T1R2 and T1R3, found in most mammals, that have evolved over millions of years in ancestral environments with a limited availability of sugars (think Paleo).[13] The excessive stimulation of your sweetness receptors by sugar-rich foods in today's processed foods *overstimulates* the reward signal in your brain, overriding your brain's self-control mechanism. Ultimately, this leads to sugar addiction and is a major reason why it's so difficult to pass on the candies, cakes and sugary treats.

4) Lack of Sleep

Sleep plays a tremendous role in controlling satiety, appetite and insulin levels. Today, the average person gets *less than 7 hours* of sleep per night and this sleep–debt exerts serious detrimental effects on your hormones.

Ghrelin is your hunger hormone, stimulating your appetite and telling your body to feed it. A high-carbohydrate meal creates a significant rise in insulin and a parallel rise in ghrelin, leaving you craving *even more* carbohydrates and simple sugars![14] Studies show that if you sleep less than seven hours per night, your ghrelin levels will significantly increase. Currently, the average person gets only 6.8 hours of sleep per night. Not surprisingly, this leads to a greater likelihood of weight gain!

The fewer hours you sleep, the greater is your production of appetite-boosting hormone ghrelin. Incredibly, even a single-night of poor sleep can strongly affect your hunger cues. A recent study found if you sleep less than five hours for a single night, you'll have markedly increased ghrelin and hunger levels.[15] Too much ghrelin causes elevated inflammatory levels and bad LDL cholesterol, decreased sex hormones and good HDL cholesterol, and increased risk of heart attack and stroke.

Ultimately, if better health or a better body is your goal, you need get at least seven hours of sleep per night. Schedule time for a quick nap in the day or simply set your alarm for later in the morning to take advantage of more time in deep, rejuvenating sleep! It's an easy, cost-effective way to reduce cravings and put the brakes on weight gain.

5) Stress

Your cortisol stress hormone and insulin blood sugar hormone have a yin-yang type of relationship. Cortisol's main role is to *raise blood sugars* so you have fuel for activity. As your blood sugars rise in response to cortisol, it results in a subsequent increase in insulin, whose role it is to get those sugars *into* the cell to be used for energy.

The problem starts when you are continually stressed because your cortisol levels will remain elevated, resulting in consistently high blood sugars and therefore consistently high insulin levels. This is a perfect recipe for weight gain and poor health.

Today, the average person is working longer hours and sleeping fewer hours than even a generation ago. Despite the benefits of the latest technology for improving work productivity and social connectivity, it has major downfalls. Most people are constantly connected via their laptops or mobile devices, which exerts a stimulatory effect on your nervous system and a constant low-grade stress on your body in the long run.

This continual sympathetic *fight or flight* stimulation raises cortisol stress hormone levels, your blood sugars and subsequently insulin levels. As previously discussed, high insulin leads to a strong addiction to sugary treats and processed snacks, exacerbating the weight-gain cycle and worsening your health. The combination of high stress (cortisol) and high insulin is something not normally seen in nature. It is a major trigger for rapid weight gain, especially around the mid-section.

INSULIN DYSFUNCTION, MOOD AND DEPRESSION

New research has uncovered the growing connection between insulin dysfunction and the increased incidence of mood disturbances and depression. In Finland, a recent study found that young men with insulin resistance were three times more likely to suffer from severe depression.[16] Peaks and valleys of insulin from excessive carb and sugar intake commonly lead to insulin resistance. Unfortunately, most people are not tested for insulin or blood sugar dysfunctions when they complain to their doctor about poor mood or depression.

In 2011, a study of over 4,000 people showed that depressive symptoms were associated with higher fasting and 30-minute insulin levels.[17] The authors made specific mention that anti-depressant medications did not alter this association, as these medications target neurotransmitters (serotonin or dopamine) and do not address blood sugar and insulin dysfunction. Other important factors associated with depression are low levels of vitamin D, zinc and testosterone.

III. THE PALEO PROJECT—INSULIN PLAN

STEP A: SELF-ASSESSMENT

Complete the *Insulin* self-assessment below and refer to the *Insulin Action Plan* table listed in Figure 7.4 for your corresponding insulin solution.

Insulin Self-Assessment

- Do you crave sweets?

- Do you get irritable, anxious or jittery if you miss a meal?

- Do you get tired a few hours after eating?

- Do you carry extra-weight around your belly?

- Do you retain water or seem sensitive to salt?

- Do you eat a high-carbohydrate breakfast (cereal, bagel, muffins, etc.)?

- Do you consume more than five units of alcohol per week?

- Do you frequently feel moody or impatient?

- Do you have type-II diabetes, high blood pressure or polycystic ovaries (PCOS)?

- Do you have chronic fungal infections (jock itch, vaginal yeast, dry scaly patches on the skin)?

STEP A: SELF-ASSESSMENT		STEP B: HACK YOUR HEALTH	STEP C: INSULIN SOLUTIONS		
Grade	Score	Lab Testing	Level 1 (Diet)	Level 2 (Alpha-Lipoic Acid)	Level 3 (Berberine)
Pass	0-2	n/a	✔	n/a	n/a
Possible Deficiency	3-5	✔	✔	✔	n/a
Support Required	6+	✔	✔	✔	✔

Figure 7.4. Insulin Action Plan

STEP B: HACK YOUR HEALTH (LAB TESTING)

All of the following lab tests should be performed if you score "possible deficiency" or "support required." They should be retested quarterly until you achieve the desired range.

Fasting Insulin

This test requires you to fast for 12 hours, typically overnight. Eat your last meal no later than 8 p.m. the night before and do not eat anything upon rising until your blood is drawn at a laboratory. Optimal values for fasting insulin are less than 40pmol/L, although normal ranges can extend all the way up to 180pmol/L.

Hemoglobin A1c (HA1c)

This test is a three-month average measure of your blood sugar levels. If test results are high then poor insulin sensitivity may be present. Optimal levels are approximately 0.048-0.054 (Canada and USA), although normal ranges typically run from 0.040-0.060.[18]

Fructoseamine

A three-week average of your blood sugar levels, fructoseamine is a shorter-term measure of your blood sugar levels. The desired range is 180-223 umol/L.

GGT (Liver Enzyme)

A liver enzyme associated with fatty liver disease, GGT is associated with insulin resistance and blood sugar dysfunction. The desired range is less than 30 U/L.[18]

CRP-hs

CRP is a measure of overall systemic inflammation. Typically, the more overweight you are, the greater your inflammatory levels. The desired range is less than 0.8 mg/L.[18]

STEP C: INSULIN SOLUTIONS

The scientific research is clear. The best ways to correct your blood sugar and insulin dysfunctions are diet and exercise. By adopting a Modern Paleo dietary approach and incorporating the right mix of exercise, you can restore insulin balance and set yourself up for successful long-term weight loss.

Level 1 Solution: The Paleo Diet and Exercise

The Paleo Diet

In Section I on Nutrition, I discussed the many health benefits of an ancestral or Paleo diet. The research shows that a Paleo diet can be a powerful weapon in preventing blood sugar and insulin dysfunction, as well as the development of diabetes, one of the most costly conditions to treat in the healthcare system.

In Sweden, a recent study compared the effects of the Paleo diet versus the standard medical diabetes diet on patients with type-2 diabetes who were taking medications for blood-sugar control. After three months, *diabetic patients on the Paleo diet had lower levels of HA1c, triglycerides, blood pressure, weight and waist circumference, as well as increased good HDL cholesterol.*[19] These are incredible changes! Consider that every 1% decrease in HA1c value correlates to an 18% decreased risk of coronary heart disease and/or stroke.[20] This has a tremendous impact on your general health and longevity.

Even the *Mediterranean diet,* long heralded as the gold standard of diets by doctors for its ability to reduce risk factors of chronic diseases, could not outperform the Paleo diet. A recent study in patients with type-2 diabetes found blood-sugar control was superior in the Paleo group compared to the Mediterranean diet group.[21] These improvements were independent of weight loss!

How long does it take to see benefits? A study at the *University of California* demonstrated that after only two weeks on the Paleo diet subjects displayed considerable reductions in insulin levels, blood pressure, total and bad LDL cholesterol, and triglycerides.[22] You will not get better or faster results with any other dietary strategy.

The emphasis of a Paleo diet on greater intakes of quality proteins and healthy fats helps to lower the glycemic index of your meal and promote better insulin balance, making you feel full for a longer stretches during the day. The emphasis on protein blunts ghrelin release, reducing hunger cravings.

The Paleo diet focuses on a higher consumption of fruits and vegetables, increasing your intake of important vitamins and minerals—namely chromium, vitamin B3 (niacin), and magnesium—all of which help to balance blood sugars. The Paleo diet is rich in soluble fibre, which slows the release of sugars absorbed in the blood, leading to sustained energy through the day. Refer to Section I for a description of all the suggested foods.

Exercise—Strength Training and Cardio
Strength training is an absolute must if you are trying to improve your health, lose weight, fit into a smaller dress or pant size, or to take your athletic potential to the next level. It's a major weapon in improving insulin sensitivity and up-regulating the GLUT-4 receptors in your muscle tissue to help soak up carbohydrates and replenish muscle glycogen stores.

The medical journal *Diabetes Care* (2013) noted the tremendous power of weight training in improving insulin resistance. The 12-month study found major improvements in insulin sensitivity and blood sugars (HA1c) in older adults with type-2 diabetes who lifted weights versus those who did not.[23] The participants also lost body fat and increased their lean muscle mass!

As for cardiovascular training, steady-state cardio helps to promote healthy blood sugar control and weight loss, but unfortunately many people don't have an extra hour or two in their day. Not to worry, there is an alternative that is an even more efficient! Short intense exercise bouts or high intensity interval training (HIIT) for 30- to 60-second intervals, interspersed with 60-second rest periods, yielded dramatic reductions in blood sugar response after only one training session.[24] Be efficient with your training and implement short intense training bouts (HIIT) to enhance your blood sugar control and weight loss progress (see Appendix B— Beginner HIIT).

Level 2 Solution: Cinnamon and Alpha-Lipoic Acid

Cinnamon

One of the oldest spices in the world, cinnamon dates to 2,700BC in Chinese medical texts. It was so highly regarded over the centuries that at one time it was considered more precious than gold.

Cinnamon deserves gold-star status for its ability to improve blood-sugar levels. Studies have shown that a 1g dose of cinnamon daily is enough to decrease fasting glucose 18-29% and improve insulin signalling.[25, 26] These improvements translate to inches off your hips and waistline.

In China, patients with type-II diabetes supplementing with cinnamon daily for three months showed remarkable reductions in their HA1c levels.[27] Better HA1c balance reflects better blood-sugar levels and therefore better insulin control. Cinnamon also helps to promote healthy cholesterol balance, lowering triglycerides, total and bad LDL cholesterol.[25] Try adding 1g of cinnamon to your protein shake or in your morning yogurt daily to enjoy these benefits.

Alpha-Lipoic Acid

A primary nutrient required for regulating insulin function, alpha-lipoic acid (ALA) improves the efficiency of insulin signalling pathways and your insulin sensitivity.[28] It's thought that the ability of ALA to improve insulin sensitivity has to do with its effect in mitigating oxidative stress and inflammation.[29]

ALA is considered the universal antioxidant because it is both fat-soluble and water-soluble, making it beneficial in both your bloodstream and in your cells. Additionally, it helps to recycle other antioxidants such as vitamin C and glutathione so they can provide even more antioxidant protection to the body. It is also a good choice for reducing inflammation, lowering bad LDL cholesterol and triglycerides, while increasing good HDL cholesterol.[30, 31]

Alpha-lipoic acid is found in red meat (grass-fed highly recommended), organ meats and brewer's yeast. You can supplement with ALA to achieve higher doses and assist in insulin balance and therefore weight loss. The recommend daily dose is 600mg; make sure to take it with food.

Level 3 Solution: Berberine

Ground-breaking new research has uncovered that *berberine* is tremendously effective at balancing blood sugar levels. It's so transformative that it has been labelled a "natural anti-diabetic drug."

A recent study compared the use of berberine supplementation versus metformin—the most commonly prescribed anti-diabetic drug—over a three-month period in type-II diabetes patients. Incredibly, berberine lowered fasting blood sugars, HA1c and insulin levels *just as well as* metformin.[32, 33] These results are remarkable! Berberine is a highly effective alternative to medications for treating blood sugar and insulin levels.

In previous chapters, I discussed berberine's beneficial impact on your digestive and immune systems. Traditionally, medicinal herbs such as goldenseal that contain strong concentrations of berberine have been used to treat intestinal ailments due to its antimicrobial properties. It is also wonderful for reducing inflammation, notoriously high in people who are overweight and obese.[34, 35] Berberine's ability to influence multiple levels of the *Paleo Project Pyramid* make it a powerful weapon in restoring optimal health and performance.

The daily recommendation is 200-300mg three times with food. Note: If taken for longer than four weeks, you should be monitored by a naturopath or other healthcare professionals.

CASE STUDY—INSULIN

Glen, a 55-year-old salesman, had been struggling with weight gain, high blood pressure, and high cholesterol for many years when he first came to see me. His doctor had given him repeated warnings to lose weight and eat better, but Glen struggled to make any positive changes. During his last visit, the doctor told him he was a "ticking time bomb" and insisted he needed to start making some changes or he would have to put him on medications.

Glen weighed 330lb (at 6' tall) and struggled with low energy levels, heartburn, bloating and sleep apnea. He was always eating out at fast food restaurants, had little time for exercise or activity (softball once weekly), suffered from chronic low back pain and confessed his libido was almost non-existent. His blood pressure was 148/92mmHg and his waist circumference 55 inches. His lab tests revealed the following results shown in Figure 7.5.

Lab Test	Normal Range	Glen's Levels	Significance
CRP-hs	Less than 1.0	6.3	Very high – reflects systemic inflammation
Fasting Insulin	Desired less than 50	100	High normal – sign of insulin insensitivity
HA1c	Desired less than 0.55	0.65	High blood sugar levels over past 3 months
Fructoseamine	Desired less than 180	320	Sign of high blood sugars over past 3 weeks
Triglycerides	Optimal less than 1.0	1.83	High – associated with poor insulin sensitivity
GGT	Less than 30	60	Very high – associated with poor insulin sensitivity

Figure 7.5. Summary of Glen's Lab Test Results

Glen's excessive weight gain over the years had resulted in systemic inflammation, a fatty liver, very high belly-fat, small intestinal bacterial overgrowth (SIBO) and high-risk factors for heart attack or stroke. He admitted he had let his weight gain spiral out of control.

When Glen came to me and said his wife and daughters had recently sat him down for an intervention-type talk, he knew the problem was reaching a tipping point. In an attempt to capitalize on his new commitment, I immediately put him on a low-carb Paleo diet, removed all sugars, processed and fast foods, as well as alcohol and caffeine. Glen struggled in the first week but stuck with the program.

I added a probiotic supplement to support gut flora, berberine to manage his blood sugars and control inflammation, and fish oils to correct for deficiencies. After the first week, he started to turn the corner as his heartburn decreased dramatically and his bloating subsided.

Finally, I provided Glen with a strength-training program (twice weekly) and cardio regimen (walking five nights of the week for 30 minutes after dinner) to get Glen's blood sugars and insulin back under control.

After four weeks, he dropped 15 pounds and his blood pressure fell to 138/88mmHg. By eight weeks he had lost another 10 pounds and his gas, bloating and heartburn symptoms were completely gone. His improved digestion and fitness level translated to better energy as well as an increase in libido (which Glen noted gave him motivation to stick with the plan!).

Finally, after 12 weeks Glen had lost another 13 pounds (38lb total), cut his CRP inflammatory levels in half and reduced his blood pressure even further to 132/86mmHg. His doctor was so impressed with the changes that he held off on prescribing medication and agreed Glen should continue for another six months following his regimen. Glen is a testament to the fact that clients who are motivated and compliant can achieve amazing results!

CHAPTER 8

CORTISOL—The Athlete's Accelerator

Have you heard the story of the ancient Greek wrestler, Milo? Around 6,000BC, Milo was considered the greatest athlete in ancient Greece. He was said to have acquired his impressive strength and physique from his early childhood, when he began carrying a baby calf, on his back, up the neighbouring mountain. He repeated this task every day, and as the calf grew heavier, Milo grew stronger. Eventually, the calf grew into a full-grown bull and Milo was still capable of lifting and carrying the massive animal up the mountain.

In today's world, stress still provides the mental and physical challenges required to stimulate positive adaptation, triggering the body to grow stronger in the process. Yes, stress can actually be good for you!

Stress is essential for overall health. Stress provides the mental and physical challenges required to make you smarter, stronger and more productive. For Milo, constantly lifting a progressively heavier load triggered a tremendous adaptive stress response, which resulted in phenomenal strength! This principle still applies today: exercise is a stress from which you grow stronger; work is a stress from which you become more productive.

Throughout our evolution, stressors would have presented themselves in many different forms—being chased by a wild animal, crossing a dangerous river or trying to hunt for your next meal. In response to these stressful stimuli, your body produces two very important catabolic hormones, cortisol and adrenaline, that allow you to react quickly and adapt to new stimuli.

This heightened state of being allows you to overcome obstacles that, in your normal state, you would not be able to conquer. Your body's hormonal stress response evolved to cope with acute events—not the daily grind of heavy traffic, never-ending emails and constantly being on the run.

Did you know that the reason for four out of every five visits to the doctor's office is stress-related? Absences from work due to stress cost employers a whopping $3.5 billion annually! Some of the most common complaints from clients are feeling rundown, having dark circles under their eyes and sleep disruptions. This constant stress ravages your hormonal survival system and creates a major roadblock in your quest for better health, weight loss and superior performance.

What exactly is stress and how can you use it to your benefit rather than to your detriment?

I. BACK TO BASICS—CORTISOL AND ADRENALINE 101

What is Stress?

The classic definition of stress is a *specific response* to a stimulus that disrupts your body's normal balance. Your body is always striving to achieve balance or *homeostasis*; however, life stressors are continually pulling you away from this state.

Stress can come in many different forms: *mental stress* from a busy work day or trying to meet deadlines, *emotional stress* from relationships with family or friends, or *physical stress* from an intense training session or constantly being on the run.

Hormesis is the term used to describe a positive adaptation to stressful stimuli. You are stressed, you grow stronger (mentally, emotionally or physically) and you thrive. This good stress or *eustress* makes you more productive at work and stronger in the gym and keeps you motivated for new adventures in life. The key factor is all about the dose. *How much* stress are you getting every day and *how intense* are the stressors?

When a stressor becomes too intense or too frequent, your body must work harder to keep up the accelerated pace. This stress eventually leads to fatigue, weight gain, cognitive decline and poor performance. If you want to build a sharper mind and leaner body, and perform well at work or in the gym, you need to understand how cortisol and adrenaline affect your body. Take a look at the physiology of stress.

Cortisol, Adrenaline and Your Adrenal Glands

Your adrenal glands are small triangular-shaped hats that sit atop your kidneys. Their role is to secrete hormones in response to stressful stimuli. Your adrenal glands allow you to adapt to stress. They are made up of two parts: the inner *medulla* and the outer *cortex*, shown in Figure 8.1. Each part performs a separate function in response to stress, so you can think of them as two separate organs.

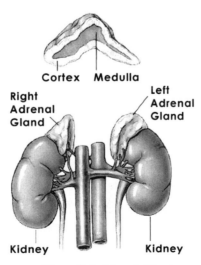

Figure 8.1. Adrenal Glands

The *inner medulla* of your adrenal glands is responsible for producing the hormone *adrenaline* in response to stress. This is your body's famous fight or flight survival response.

Imagine you hear a strange noise at night and think there is burglar in your house. Instantly, your heart starts racing and your brain sends a direct message to the inner medulla of your adrenal glands to produce *adrenaline*, your body's survival switch!

Adrenaline acts by increasing your blood pressure, shunting blood to your muscles, dilating your pupils, pumping your heart and lungs faster, and increasing your blood sugars to provide fuel for the fight or flight moment. All of these actions happen instantly via your *sympathetic* fight or flight nervous system, a direct connection between your brain and adrenal glands.

During this fight or flight moment, the adrenal cortex receives an important message from your brain to produce cortisol. Cortisol is classified as a glucocorticoid and its main role is to increase your blood-sugar levels by stimulating the breakdown of lean muscle and glycogen for fuel.

Here is how it works. The hypothalamus area of your brain, the master hormone conductor, tells your pituitary gland to produce adreno-corticotrophin hormone (ACTH), seen in Figure 8.2, which then travels down to your adrenal glands to stimulate cortisol production. This is a *slower and more sustained* response to stress, as ACTH must travel through your bloodstream.

The outer cortex of your adrenal glands produces another important hormone called *dehydroepiandrostenedione* (DHEA). DHEA is a powerful anabolic hormone that is a precursor for the sex hormones testosterone and estrogen. It serves as an important marker of stress and plays a critical role in liver, immune and brain function.

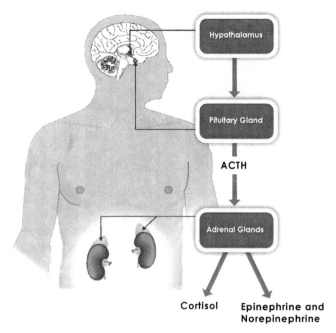

Figure 8.2. HPA-Axis Summary

Your Cortisol Rhythm

Normal functioning adrenal glands secrete small and precise amounts of cortisol through the day. In the morning, cortisol levels should be at their highest in order to wake you from your deep sleep, increase your alertness and prepare you for the day ahead. If you struggle to wake up in the morning, hit the snooze button multiple times or need a caffeine boost to get yourself moving then chances are you have *low morning cortisol* levels. This type of abnormal cortisol rhythm can cause fatigue, poor memory, inability to concentrate, irritability and lack of productivity during the day.

As the day progresses, your cortisol levels should naturally decline and reach their lowest point around bedtime. This decrease in cortisol allows your sleep hormone *melatonin* to ramp up, triggering deep and restful sleep. Melatonin reaches peak levels in the blood several hours after you fall asleep, which then stimulates the production of growth hormone (GH).

Growth hormone is your body's fountain of youth hormone that promotes lean muscle, superior recovery, strong libido and positive mood. If you are a night owl and get a burst of energy before bed, you may have high evening cortisol levels. This can suppress your natural production of melatonin and limit your GH output overnight. If you've been training too frequently or too intensely, you may experience trouble falling asleep. This type of abnormal cortisol rhythm leads to fatigue during the day (waking is adequate but you are not well rested), feeling "tired but wired" and difficulty falling asleep at night.

The Original Stress Theory: General Adaptation Syndrome

During the period of writing this book, a major shift has been made in terms of how we understand stress. Until now, expert researchers have based their recommendations on the *General Adaptation Syndrome* theory of stress—a theory that has remained strong since 1936. However, a new branch of medicine called *psycho-neuro-endocrine immunology (PNEI)* has changed the way we think about dealing with stress by uncovering amazing connections between your brain's command centre and adrenal dysfunction. Let me explain.

In 1936, a renowned Hungarian scientist named Hans Selye wrote an article in the British journal *Nature* describing how animals and humans adapt to stressors in their environment. His theory was called the *General Adaptation Syndrome* and consisted of three distinct stages (see Figure 8.3).

The first stage is called the *alarm reaction phase*, when your body produces adrenaline to provide you with a quick boost for the upcoming fight or flight moment during a one-rep maximum squat or a new deadline at work. This amount of stimulation cannot be sustained for long periods and is characterized by elevated cortisol and DHEA levels. Adverse symptoms are typically not prevalent at this stage but can include some mild fatigue.

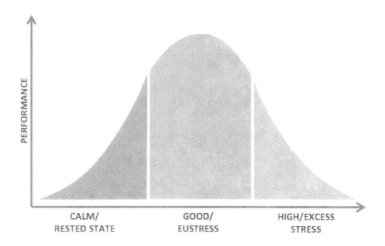

PERFORMANCE

CALM/
RESTED STATE

GOOD/
EUSTRESS

HIGH/EXCESS
STRESS

Figure 8.3. General Adaptation Syndrome

The second stage of adaptation is called the *resistance phase*, when your body adapts to the stressors by producing greater amounts of cortisol. High cortisol and low DHEA levels characterize the resistance phase, the result of increased use of the hormone *pregnenolone* to produce more cortisol at the expense of DHEA. Your body can sustain this output only for a limited time before it succumbs to the stressors.

The third stage is called the *exhaustion phase*, the point at which your body can no longer cope with the stressors. You have pushed your body and adrenal glands to the edge and they can no longer keep up. This is when you feel burn out or *adrenal exhaustion*, characterized by low levels of *both* cortisol and DHEA.

The Original Stress Theory gives you a general understanding of how stress affects the body; however, it is *not* the whole story. New research provides a clearer understanding of how stress affects us from many different angles. Take a look at this section.

The New Stress Theory: Adrenal Dysfunction

A new branch of medicine called *psycho-neuro-endocrine immunology (PNEI)* is shifting the landscape of how we view stress and adrenal dysfunction. PNEI is uncovering connections between your brain's command centre, which is the hypothalamus, and important systems of the body: your nervous system, hormonal system and immune system.

These systems are constantly providing feedback to your brain, which assesses the incoming information and relays the message to your adrenal glands. What messages is it relaying? These messages come in many different chemical forms: *neurotransmitters* from your nervous system, *cytokines* from your immune system and *hormones* from your sex organs (testes and ovaries) and adrenal glands.

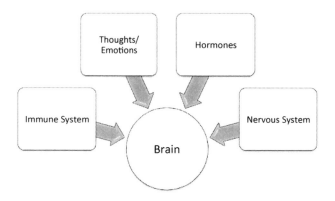

Figure 8.4. Summary of PNEI Stress Response

This new area of medicine suggests the adrenal glands are not so much fatigued but rather stuck in overdrive or stuck in the mud (sluggish), simply doing what they are told by your brain. This relationship is shown in Figure 8.4.

To simplify things, you can think of the messages from your brain to the adrenal glands as two distinct groups: *stimulatory* signals or *inhibitory* signals. If your hypothalamus receives more stimulating signals than inhibitory, it will lead to greater output of cortisol and adrenaline from your adrenal glands. This leads to trouble falling asleep, feeling "tired but wired" during the day and having poor immunity.

On the other hand, if your body receives greater inhibitory signals than stimulating ones, your adrenal glands will be sluggish and produce decreased amounts cortisol and adrenaline. This leaves you struggling to wake up in the morning, feeling tired all day long or having difficulty staying asleep through the night. Later in this chapter, you will see the most common scenarios occurring in clinical practice and learn to identify the pattern of adrenal dysfunction that applies to you.

Just like the firing pattern of your muscles, your body has preferred firing patterns for biochemical pathways that adapt to stress. Program the correct responses and you'll adapt successfully. Remain stuck in poor reactive pathways and you'll struggle to keep up.

Negative Effects of Adrenal Dysfunction
The negative effects of chronic stress, altered hypothalamic function and adrenal dysfunction are well documented. You can see a list of the detrimental effects of high stress levels in Figure 8.5.

Negative Effects of Adrenal Dysfunction
• Increases inflammation (TNF-alpha, IL-1, Th1 immune response)
• Reduces acetylcholine production, resulting in poor memory
• Increases likelihood for anxiety and depression
• Damages the hippocampus, resulting in short-term memory loss
• Reduces serotonin levels, the body's precursor to the sleep hormone melatonin
• Lowers growth hormone (GH), the body's *fountain of youth* hormone
• Reduces deep, rejuvenating sleep
• Increases abdominal circumference and visceral belly-fat
• Inhibits thyroid function, thereby slowing metabolism
• Promotes insulin resistance
• Leads to loss of lean muscle tissue
• Leads to cognitive decline

Figure 8.5. Summary of Negative Effects of Adrenal Dysfunction

CORTISOL AND WEIGHT GAIN

Stress has a major connection to weight gain. Cortisol blocks the release of your satiety hormone leptin from fat cells and dramatically impairs your ability to burn fat. The negative impact of cortisol on weight gain doesn't end there.

In Chapter 6, I discussed how brown fat can be burned readily for fuel, while white fat sticks more easily to the body and is more harmful to overall health. New research shows that cortisol inhibits a key enzyme called PGC1-alpha, normally produced during exercise that converts white fat to brown fat.[1] More white fat means you will have a harder time losing weight and shedding excess body fat. In short, stress can literally make you fat!

II. HOW THINGS GO WRONG—CORTISOL DYSFUNCTION

Figure 8.6 is a comprehensive list of the various factors that may affect your adrenal health. Individually or in combination, these factors may contribute to *adrenal dysfunction* and sabotage your quest to trim your waistline, achieve a new personal best race time or improve your general health.

Adrenals: Summary of How Things Go Wrong	
Diet	Insufficient protein intake
	Insufficient or excessive carbohydrate intake
	Insufficient or imbalanced intake of fats
	Excessive alcohol consumption
	Dehydration
	Methylxanthines – caffeine, tea, chocolate
Digestion	Intestinal dysbiosis
	Leaky gut
	Food allergies
Immunity	Depressed immunity
	Infections – virus, bacteria, fungus, parasite
	Low sIgA
	Th1 & Th2 imbalance
Inflammation	Elevated CRP levels
	Elevated ESR levels
	Cytokine storm
Hormones	Blood sugar surges
	Poor sleep
	Stress – mental, physical, emotional
Training	Overtraining
	Depleted glycogen stores
	Excessive muscle damage
Other	Toxic heavy metals
	Anemia
	Radiation
	Traumatic event

Figure 8.6. Summary of How Things Go Wrong

To simplify this complex picture, look at the four most common causes of adrenal dysfunction seen in clinical practice:

1. Too Many Stimulants (Caffeine!)

2. Too Much Stress

3. Too Many Carbs

4. Not Enough Sleep

I) Too Many Stimulants

Coffee is one of the world's most popular beverages, providing a natural boost in mood, work capacity and mental focus. The caffeine in your morning cup of coffee helps to increase fat burning while sparing precious lean muscle and it delays fatigue during exercise. While coffee can be beneficial to your health, it can also be a serious detriment. You can get too much of a good thing!

Caffeine is a central nervous system stimulant that blocks the release of adenosine, a neurotransmitter with a calming effect on the body. This results in the release of adrenaline from your adrenals and activation of your fight or flight sympathetic nervous system. Caffeine is what gives you that extra boost in the morning, before a big workout or when you are trying to meet deadlines at work.

Caffeine stimulates the release of *dopamine*, the body's feel-good neurotransmitter that activates the pleasure centres of the brain. Dopamine perks up your mood, increases mental focus and allows you to be in the zone during work or training.

So, what's the problem with drinking a lot of coffee? Well, there are numerous risks associated with an elevated caffeine intake. The excessive adrenaline release may leave you stuck in a sympathetic overdrive with symptoms of restlessness, headache, irritability and poor recovery. Much like alcohol, you build up a tolerance to caffeine, which means you need greater and greater quantities to stimulate the same response. This has diminishing returns in the long term and is the perfect recipe for adrenal dysfunction and fatigue.

Caffeine is also a diuretic, promoting the loss of fluids from the body and increased likelihood of dehydration with excessive intake. Remember, dehydration is an absolute performance killer that can impair your digestion and immunity as well as increase stress hormone levels.

Finally, most people don't realize that the *half-life* of caffeine is six hours, which means if you drink your last cup of coffee (400mg of caffeine) at 2 p.m., you will still have 200mg of caffeine in your bloodstream at

8 p.m., and incredibly still 100mg of caffeine in your bloodstream at 2 a.m.! This can sabotage your deep sleep, blunt growth-hormone release and lead to fatigue and poor recovery.

2) Too Much Stress

Stress can literally make you fat. Dr. Michael Schwartz at the *University of Washington* showed that individuals who were overweight had marked changes in the hypothalamus area of their brains. His research suggests these changes alter the way your brain relays messages via your HPA-axis. It plays a much greater role in weight gain versus total calories consumed.[2] Stress initiates a hormonal cascade that leaves you craving sugars and stuck in fat-building mode.

Being overweight or obese inhibits the production of new nerve cells in your hypothalamus, adding credence to the notion that damage to this area of the brain may impair your HPA-axis, alter adrenal output and contribute strongly to weight gain.[3]

If this theory holds true, it would be possible to achieve critical weight loss only with stress-reduction protocols. A compelling new study of 2,800 people showed that stress management programs in the work-place resulted in greater weight loss compared to only dietary changes.[4] This is a very important finding. Without changing diet or exercise habits, researchers were able to trigger significant weight loss via just breathing and stress-management techniques.

3) Too Many Carbs

When you combine high stress levels with a high carbohydrate diet, you have the perfect recipe for rapid weight gain, especially around the mid-section. Chronically high cortisol levels lead to consistently elevated blood sugars, eventually impairing your insulin sensitivity or ability to process carbohydrates. This means your body needs to produce more insulin to cope with a high-carbohydrate diet.

Cortisol affects your brain, activating reward centres that cause strong cravings and neuropeptides (NPY) that increase your appetite for sugary and fatty foods. It can quickly become a downward spiral. High stress leads to strong cravings for sugar and increased appetite, which leads to the overconsumption of sugars and carbs, followed by weight gain and increasing cortisol stress levels. In order to regain control, you need to improve your stress response. Solutions are given at the end of this chapter.

4) Not Enough Sleep

In the Paleolithic hunter-gatherer era, our ancestors woke with the rising sun in the morning and rested their heads for a good night's sleep not long after sundown. Scientists have estimated they averaged about ten hours of sleep per night.[5] The absence of external light sources, televisions, laptops and mobile devices made it a lot easier to get to bed early but the benefits are deeply engrained in your DNA.

Your circadian rhythms are based on the light and dark cycles of the day and they have a profound effect on your ability to burn fat, on your athletic performance and your health.

Two generations ago, your grandparents averaged 9-10 hours of sleep per night, not far off our Paleolithic ancestors. Today, the average North American gets about 6.5 hours of sleep per night, about an hour or two less than the recommended 7.0 to 8.5 hours of sleep. You can see this trend in Figure 8.7. Over the course of a year this amounts to approximately a 500-hour sleep debt!

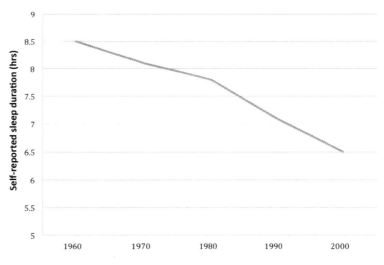

Figure 8.7. Total Sleep Time Over Last 50 Years

Sleep loss quickly throws off your cortisol levels and leads to adrenal dysfunction. Studies show that reduced sleep time leads to an altered cortisol rhythm the following day and to a reduced ability to cope with stress.[6] The medical journal *Sleep Medicine* concluded that average sleep times have decreased considerably in the last 50 years and the repercussions are altered sympathetic nervous system activity, increased cortisol output and decreased growth hormone.[7]

We all suffer from lack of sleep from time to time. Whether it's from business travel, raising children or simply working long hours into the night, everyone can cope with periods of reduced sleep. The key is not to make it a habit. The research is clear—a lack of sleep is an absolute performance killer and is strongly associated with increased appetite and weight gain.

PATTERNS OF ADRENAL DYSFUNCTION

The three most common scenarios seen in clinical practice are: cortisol rhythm dysfunction, underperforming adrenals and over-performing adrenals.

Cortisol Rhythm Dysfunction

The *hippocampus* area in your brain is responsible for controlling your natural daily cortisol rhythms described earlier in this chapter. When this rhythm gets disrupted, you may struggle with fatigue, poor memory, sleep disturbances and poor recovery.

The hippocampus is responsible for converting short-term memory to long-term memory. If you've ever struggled to remember a client's name, what you need to pick up at the grocery store or where you put your car keys, chances are you are experiencing these effects first hand. High levels of cortisol damage the hippocampus, which leads to poor short-term memory, depression and even dementia.[8, 9] See the full list of symptoms of cortisol rhythm dysfunction in Figure 8.8.

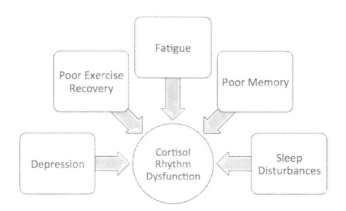

Figure 8.8. Key Symptoms of "Cortisol Rhythm Dysfunction"

Underperforming Adrenals

If you struggle to wake up in the morning, have low energy throughout the day, feel better after eating meals or have low libido, then chances are your adrenal glands are underperforming. When stress becomes long term or the accumulation of inhibitory signals to your brain exceeds the stimulatory ones, your adrenal output will tend to decline.

This is commonly seen in type-A people, typically executives, entrepreneurs and high achievers whose jobs require long working hours, endurance athletes training for a competition, or busy parents trying to balance the commitments of work and family life.

Sluggish adrenal gland function can lead to poor focus and concentration, lack of productivity, slow recovery and irritability throughout the day. Another common symptom of *underperforming* adrenals is *orthostatic hypotension* or a feeling of light-headedness when going from lying down to standing up.

The *underperforming* adrenal picture will often leave you searching for a caffeine hit or sugary snack in the morning or mid-afternoon to give yourself an artificial boost. While you may get temporary relief, it will worsen the situation in the long term. The underperforming adrenal client will commonly experience increased likelihood of colds and flu and a tendency toward low blood sugars and increased inflammation. Symptoms are shown in Figure 8.9.

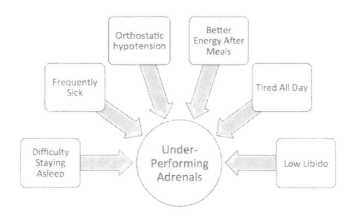

Figure 8.9. Key Symptoms of Underperforming Adrenals

Over-performing Adrenals

Over-performing adrenals occur when you feel stuck in overdrive, your mind continually racing with the list of tasks and deadlines you need to meet. This constant fight or flight sympathetic dominance chronically elevates cortisol levels and may lead to roadblocks in your quest for a slimmer waistline, faster 10k run time or better overall health.

Laptops, cellphones and exposure to WiFi are all necessary to be productive at work but they stimulate your nervous system. Spending too much time in this fight or flight mode is like hitting the accelerator of your car too frequently—it will eventually burn out your engine.

If your goal is to shed body fat, this can be problematic because the primary role of cortisol is to increase blood sugars. As blood sugars rise to meet your body's fuel demands, so do your insulin levels. Remember, high insulin levels inhibit fat loss by blocking your fat-burning enzyme (HSL).

In terms of athletic performance, elevated cortisol reduces your testosterone levels and limits your ability to build lean muscle mass. It does so by inhibiting your pituitary gland's production of *leutinizing hormone (LH)*, which acts directly on the testes or ovaries to produce testosterone. When your stress levels rise, you reduce the LH signal to the sex organs (testes and ovaries) and subsequently reduce your testosterone output.

Chronically high cortisol depletes secretory IgA levels, leaving your first line of immune defence more susceptible to colds and flu. It decreases frontal lobe activity in your brain, impairing your ability to concentrate and maintain mental clarity. It's not the ideal scenario if you need to be sharp at work.

Finally, if you suffer from over-performing adrenals, you may have difficulty falling asleep at night. If you characterize yourself as a night owl or do your best work late into the night, this may be you! Elevated evening cortisol due to over-performing adrenals may suppress deep sleep, melatonin production and ultimately your precious growth hormone production at night. Symptoms are shown in Figure 8.10.

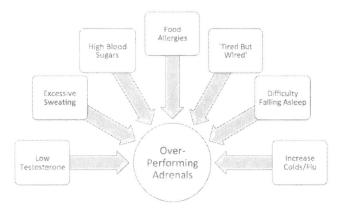

Figure 8.10. Symptoms of Over-Performing Adrenals

III. THE PALEO PROJECT—CORTISOL PLAN

STEP A: SELF-ASSESSMENT

Fill out the *Cortisol* self-assessment and implement the corresponding *Cortisol Action Plan* from the chart in Figure 8.11.

Cortisol Self-Assessment

- Do you have low blood pressure or ever feel dizzy when you stand up?

- Do you crave salt or sweets?

- Do you have dark circles under your eyes?

- Do you have sleep disturbances (trouble falling asleep or staying asleep)?

- Do you have feel sluggish first thing in the morning?

- Do you consume two or more cups of coffee per day?

- Do you have poor tolerance to alcohol, caffeine or other drugs?

- Do you feel busy or stressed most of the time?

- Do you have anxiety, heart palpitations or suffer from panic attacks?

- Do you have mental fogginess or trouble concentrating?

STEP A: SELF-ASSESSMENT		STEP B: HACK YOUR HEALTH	STEP C: CORTISOL SOLUTIONS		
Grade	Score	Lab Testing	Level 1 (Diet & Breathwork)	Level 2 (Alpha-GPC + PS)	Level 3 (Rhodiola + Ginseng or Withania)
Pass	0-2	n/a	✔	n/a	n/a
Possible Deficiency	3-5	✔	✔	✔	n/a
Support Required	6+	✔	✔	✔	✔

Figure 8.11. Cortisol Action Plan

If you scored "possible deficiency," you likely have a cortisol rhythm dysfunction. If you score "support required," you may have under-performing or over-performing adrenals. A subsequent test will help identify your pattern in Step C.

STEP B: HACK YOUR HEALTH (LAB TESTING)

All of the following lab tests should be performed if you score "possible deficiency" or "support required." They should be retested quarterly until you achieve the desired ranges.

Adrenal Panel (Saliva)

To assess adrenal function, readings must be obtained at multiple times of the day upon rising, mid-morning, mid-afternoon and bedtime. This will determine your cortisol rhythm throughout the day. Studies show that salivary cortisol levels correlate very accurately (approximately 93%) with blood levels.[10] This test also measures salivary DHEA levels.

Cortisol and Free Testosterone (Blood)

This test is performed via blood draw at a medical laboratory as early in the morning as possible. In clinical practice, I typically test cortisol along with free testosterone, as the ratio between the two acts as a marker for overtraining and high stress.

However, there are several major drawbacks with drawing blood to test for cortisol. You obtain only a single measurement, the act of a drawing blood is stressful and labs are not open until 8 a.m., well after most people wake up in the morning. This makes the salivary adrenal panel a far superior assessment tool.

DHEA (Saliva or Blood)

DHEA levels are assessed in conjunction with cortisol in the salivary Adrenal Panel test. They can also be assessed along with the cortisol and free testosterone in a blood draw. DHEA levels are used in a ratio with cortisol to determine your stress levels. Salivary levels correlate very highly (approximately 81%) with levels found in the blood.[11]

Note: Salivary measures of testosterone and estrogen correlate very poorly with blood levels, at 22% and 32% respectively.

Physical Measurements

Physical changes associated with elevated cortisol levels are increased abdominal skinfold thickness and increased abdominal circumference. For men, a waist circumference greater than 38 inches is associated with a much greater risk of developing chronic diseases such as hypertension, high cholesterol, heart disease and diabetes. For women, chronic disease risk increases at waist circumference greater than 36 inches. Your *ideal* measurements may be significantly lower than these general health markers.

HEART RATE VARIABILITY (HRV)

Yogis have known for centuries that the breath is the connection between your mind and body. Your sympathetic fight or flight and parasympathetic rest and digest nervous systems interact continuously to maintain your heart rate and heart rhythm. Now, new technology allows you to measure your ability to recover (indicating how effectively you can turn off your sympathetic drive).

How does it work? When you inhale, your sympathetic tone increases, causing a mild increase in your heart rate. When you exhale, your sympathetic tone decreases, in conjunction with a natural increase in parasympathetic tone, resulting in a lowered heart rate. If you are over-training and your sympathetic system is over-stimulated, it will blunt your parasympathetic system and you will experience minimal variance in heart rate. In contrast, if your ability to recover is optimal, you will see a greater variance in heart rate, reflecting effective parasympathetic tone.

Studies show that decreased HRV (i.e., too stressed) is strongly associated with increased overnight cortisol levels, increased glucose levels and HA1c and increased pro-inflammatory cytokines.[12] These fluctuations in blood sugars and elevations in cortisol are commonly seen in clients with over-performing adrenals and can lead to weight gain and fat accumulation around the abdomen.

For athletes, a recent study of elite swimmers showed significant decreased HRV (increased sympathetic tone) when athletes got colds and flu.[13] Using a heart rate monitor, new technology allows you to measure the variability in your heart rate, which is the degree of change or a lack of change that can tell you if you are rested and ready to train or stressed and need a rest.

STEP C: CORTISOL SOLUTIONS
Level 1 Solution: Diet, Breath Work/Meditation and Sleep

Diet

- Increase Healthy Saturated Fats

- Increase Protein Intake

- Correct Nutrient Deficiencies (Vit C, B5, Magnesium, Sodium)

- Reduce Caffeine Intake

- <u>Caution</u> with Low-Carb Approach

In the early 1900s, doctor used to diagnose individuals with debilitating fatigue with *neuresthenia* or nervous system exhaustion. This diagnosis was very common at the time and the equivalent to today's *adrenal fatigue*. The treatment for this condition was simple—a high-fat diet!

Today, science confirms this age-old approach of treating neuresthenia or adrenal dysfunction. Healthy saturated fats in the form of ghee, butter (grass-fed is best) and coconut oil, as well as monounsaturated fats in the form of extra-virgin olive oil and avocados, has been shown to improve cortisol and sex hormone levels (testosterone and estrogen) in athletes training at high-intensity[14] (i.e., high-level endurance athletes, rigorous off-season training camps, CrossFit Games trainees). If you are busy at work, training frequently and always on the go, it's essential to include these healthy fats in your diet.

Next, consuming adequate protein is critical in maintaining optimal adrenal health. You should strive to obtain 1.5-2.0g/kg bodyweight per day in order to support adrenal health, as amino acids are needed for muscular recovery, immune health, hormonal health and nervous system support. Incorporate more Modern Paleo meals into your diet to help achieve your required intake.

High stress levels may deplete important nutrients that exacerbate your adrenal dysfunction symptoms. Vitamin C is a potent antioxidant that has been shown to reduce the cortisol response, post-training.[15]

It provides robust anti-inflammatory support to the body, so be sure to include the following foods in your diet: bell peppers, citrus fruits, cruciferous veggies, and leafy greens. Vitamin-B5 supports healthy adrenal cortex function, which is responsible for your cortisol production. Vitamin B5 is found abundantly in yogurt, avocados, mushrooms, broccoli and sweet potatoes. Finally, sodium levels fall dramatically in those with adrenal dysfunction; therefore, it's important to add sea salt or table salt to your meals to ensure an optimal sodium–potassium balance.

Caffeine is a powerful weapon in supporting weight loss and better performance. However, if your adrenals are not performing up to par, you need to take your foot off the caffeine accelerator. Start by cutting your coffee intake by 50% and ensuring your last cup is no later than noon. If you scored high on the *Cortisol* self-assessment, you should discontinue completely for two to four weeks.

Lastly, be cautious about adopting a low-carb dietary approach when you are highly stressed. Studies show that low-carb (less than 100g) or ketogenic diets (less than 50g) can exacerbate symptoms of adrenal dysfunction (particularly in females), as cortisol levels can rise rapidly and lead to excessive loss of muscle mass and slowing of the metabolism. Not ideal for weight loss or performance!

Breath Work/Meditation
Meditation is an ancient technique that affects your health and wellbeing. It helps restore adrenal health by stimulating your vagus nerve, which is responsible for increasing parasympathetic nervous system activity. Proper breathing is the stimulus that tells your body, "Relax! All is well!"

The role of your parasympathetic nervous system (PNS) is to balance out your fight or flight sympathetic system. Essentially, if you are burning the candle at both ends, your PNS builds the candle back up! By incorporating some simple breath work (meditation), you can increase the activation of your PNS and calm an over-active stress response. The key is all in your breath.

Not convinced? A recent study of medical students showed that those engaging in daily mindfulness meditation practices had much lower blood cortisol levels compared to a placebo.[16] Meditation has been shown to provide great improvements in patients with anxiety and depression, classic symptoms of chronically underperforming adrenals.[17]

Try this simple breathing exercise below. It can be performed at work, on the subway or before bed.

Breath Work (Meditation): 5-10 minutes

- Start by sitting with your eyes closed.

- Inhale deeply through your nose; let your belly expand for three seconds.

- At the end of your inhale, hold your breath for one second.

- Exhale deeply through your nose for another count of three seconds; let your belly draw inward toward your spine.

- Repeat these steps for 5-10 minutes.

Restorative Sleep

As I've discussed previously, you should aim for 7 to 8.5 hours of sleep per night to optimally restore your adrenal function and overall health. Ensure you are getting enough sleep and that the quality of sleep is good. In traditional Chinese medicine, they suggest the hours of sleep before midnight count as double, due to their powerful regenerative nature. Therefore, you should ideally be getting to bed before midnight (around 10-11 p.m.).

How can you improve your sleep quality? Here are some simple tips:

- Make sure your bedroom is completely dark. Try using blackout blinds or an eye mask to prevent unwanted light.

- Remove all stimulating light sources from your bedside table: cellphones, laptops and red lights from alarm clocks. These may stimulate your nervous system and prevent deep sleep.

- Turn down the lights in your house after 9 p.m. and shut off the television or laptop at least 45 minutes before bed to allow your body and nervous system to properly unwind.

- Keep your bedroom cool and wear loose-fitting clothing or sleep naked.

- Stay away from sleeping pills. Although they increase the duration of sleep, they do not improve the *quality* of your sleep.

Level 2 Solution: Alpha-GPC and PS

If you scored "possible deficiency" on your *Cortisol* self-assessment, you likely have cortisol rhythm dysfunction. Manage this dysfunction by supporting the hippocampus area of your brain and resetting your natural cortisol rhythm. (It's just like rebooting your computer!)

Alpha-Glycerophosphocholine (Alpha-GPC)

Today, people are overstimulated by constant connectivity to laptops, mobile devices and the increasing blurring of the lines between workdays and your personal time. The hippocampus helps to regulate your HPA-axis by supporting a healthy cortisol rhythm, characterized by higher cortisol levels upon rising and lower levels at bedtime.

Alpha-GPC plays an important role in the production of acetylcholine, a stimulatory neurotransmitter in the body typically depleted in those with busy schedules, lacking sleep or with high stress.[18] The neurons of your hippocampus require considerable amounts of acetylcholine for optimal function. Supplementing with alpha-GPC provides the hippocampus with the right building blocks to restore normal cortisol patterns.

The recommended dose is 1,000mg *upon rising* each day.

Phosphatidylserine (PS)

Phosphatidylserine (PS) is a primary building block of your cellular membranes and plays a key role in regulating your cortisol response. During times of stress or intense training your cortisol rhythm may stay elevated throughout the day and into the evening (when it should naturally be lower), disrupting your sleep hormones and ability to get good quality sleep.

This disruption of the cortisol rhythm may occur from working too hard or training too intensely, leaving you stuck in adrenal overdrive, as your cortisol levels stay elevated.

This scenario is commonly seen in endurance athletes, due to the longer nature of their training bouts and higher volume of training. A recent study at the *University of Mississippi* demonstrated the beneficial effects of supplementing with 600mg of PS following intense cycling bouts. After ten days, the cyclists showed major improvements in their testosterone to cortisol ratio when compared to a placebo.[19] PS supplementation has also been shown to improve recovery, minimize lean tissue breakdown and support healthy cognitive function.[20] Athletes undertaking highly glycolytic training where lactic acid production is elevated (e.g., CrossFit, off-season training camps, Ironman competitions) would also benefit greatly as would anyone logging long hours at work.

The recommended daily dose is 400–800mg taken *post-training* or *before bed*. Note: PS should *never* be taken before training, as low cortisol levels prior to exercise may impair performance.

Level 3 Solution: Rhodiola and Ginseng OR Withania

If your test score showed "support required" in the *Cortisol* self-assessment, you need to identify your distinct picture of adrenal dysfunction. Complete the second round *Self-Assessments* for Underperforming Adrenals and Over-Performing Adrenals. Whichever test you score highest on, implement the appropriate protocol from the *Adrenal Dysfunction Action Plan* in Figure 8.12.

Underperforming Adrenals Self-Assessment

- Do you feel tired throughout the day?

- Do you have lower than normal libido?

- Do you have difficulty staying asleep throughout the night?

- Do you frequently get sick?

- Do you feel more energy after eating meals?

- Do you have low blood pressure or feel light-headed when going from lying down to standing up?

Over-Performing Adrenals Self-Assessment

- Do you feel tired but wired throughout the day?

- Do you have lower than normal testosterone levels?

- Do you have difficulty falling asleep at bedtime?

- Do you suffer from excessive sweating?

- Do you suffer from food allergies?

- Do you have high blood sugar levels (or crave sweets)?

Self-Assessment	Insert Your Score	Which Is Your Higher Score? (Determine Your *Adrenal Action Plan*)
Underperforming Adrenals		If you **scored higher** in this self-assessment implement the *Underperforming Adrenal Solutions* (Rhodiola and Ginseng)
Over-Performing Adrenals		If you **scored higher** in this self-assessment implement the *Over-Performing Adrenal Solutions* (Withania)

Figure 8.12. Adrenal Dysfunction Action Plan

★ *If your scores are identical, implement the over-performing solution listed below.*

I) UNDERPERFORMING ADRENALS SOLUTION: RHODIOLA AND GINSENG

Native to the high altitude regions of Russia and Siberia, rhodiola is classified as an *adaptagen* herb because it has the ability to *improve your body's response to stress*. During the Cold War, rhodiola was used by soldiers in the former Soviet Union to combat the fatigue caused by training and living at high altitudes. New research confirms rhodiola's ability to support the adrenal response, prevent fatigue, enhance immunity, improve concentration and boost libido.[21, 22] It is widely used as a general tonic for increasing productivity at work.

Panax ginseng is another powerful adaptagen herb found in the mountainous regions of Korea, China and Japan. Its roots have long been used in traditional medicines for its ability to combat mental and physical exhaustion. Panax ginseng supports healthy hormone production and stimulates the nervous system, providing those who experience low vitality, exhaustion or low libido with a boost.

In combination, these two herbs are fantastic for boosting sluggish cortisol output from underperforming adrenals.

The recommended daily dose is 300-600mg rhodiola and 200-500mg ginseng. My favourite formula is the *Rhodiola & Ginseng Combo* by Mediherb. *Note:* Do not take at the same time as coffee or caffeinated drinks.

II) OVER PERFORMING ADRENALS SOLUTION: WITHANIA

Withania or ashwagandha, as it is known in its native India, is an adaptagen herb like rhodiola and ginseng but with slightly different properties. It is best suited for people who naturally have a lot of energy and might run themselves into the ground from being too busy, training too much or stuck in the "tired but wired" mode.

The plant chemicals *withanolides* give this herb its potent anti-fatigue properties, as well as calming effects that help to reduce the excessive stress response taxing your nervous system.[23]

In short, if you are burning the candle at both ends, this is the herb for you! It has been shown to reduce inflammation and enhance cognition, which means you may no longer need your caffeine boost to keep your mind sharp at work.[23] The recommended daily dose is 300–600g.

CASE STUDY—ADRENALS

Marie, a 32-year-old professional, came to me complaining of feeling burned out, struggling to get out of bed in the morning, feeling consistently tired and irritable throughout the day, and lacking motivation to exercise. Her weekly activity included CrossFit twice weekly, yoga and running. She said it had become worse over the last few years since the birth of her first child and balancing a high-stress job.

Marie managed a large team at work and said she was constantly on the phone, day and night, addressing work issues. She was a vegetarian who consumed egg whites and dairy but avoided all meat. Marie did not drink coffee but regularly used a pre-exercise supplement to give her energy for her workout and said she often struggled to stay asleep throughout the night. Her lab results are summarized in Figure 8.13.

Lab Test	Normal Range	Marie's Levels	Significance
Cortisol AM	2-11	1.8	Low – sign of under-performing adrenals
Cortisol NOON	1-7	0.8	Low – sign of under-performing adrenals
Cortisol PM	0.5-3.5	0.35	Low – sign of under-performing adrenals
Cortisol BEDTIME	0.20-1.3	0.15	Low – sign of under-performing adrenals
DHEA	1.2-8	2.0	Low – sign of moderately long-term stress response

Figure 8.13. Summary of Marie's Lab Test Results

Marie had a classic case of underperforming adrenals. To help correct this dysfunction, I made a few additions to her diet: eating three whole eggs for breakfast rather than just egg whites, adding a rice protein shake (30g) after training, increasing her saturated fat intake by adding butter to her veggies at lunch and dinner, eliminating all beans in favour of lentils, and discontinuing her pre-workout supplement (which contained 250mg of caffeine) in the afternoons.

I added some herbal supplements: rhodiola to support her adrenal function and alpha-GPC to help normalize her cortisol rhythm. Lastly, I made sure Marie turned off her phone at least an hour before she went to bed and I asked her to perform 15 minutes of deep breathing before bedtime to promote deeper sleep.

Marie was a little nervous about seemingly "eating so much" and increasing her fat intake. I encouraged her to give it a try for four weeks and then see how she felt. After the first week, she emailed me and said her mood had lifted and she felt less irritable at work. After two weeks, Marie commented that she was sleeping through the night for the first time in a long time. Finally, two months into the protocol, Marie's energy and enthusiasm had fully returned. She was thriving at work, enjoying her CrossFit training, and keeping up with her little boy around the house.

SECTION III

Achieve Your Potential

"The will to win, the desire to succeed, the urge to reach your full potential ...
these are the keys that will unlock the door to personal excellence."
~*Confucius*

You've now arrived at the peak of the *Paleo Project Pyramid*. Over the last eight chapters you've laid the foundation for better health and performance by upgrading your nutrition via a Modern Paleo diet and correcting imbalances and deficiencies in your body by hacking your health. Your body is now running on all cylinders. It's time to build on this foundation and take your journey to better health, a better body and better performance to the next level.

In Section III, I've developed two platforms to allow you to achieve your primary goal: fat loss/body composition or performance. It's very important for you to clearly define the direction that you want to take. While you can make progress trying to achieve both goals at the same time, you'll make the *most* progress by focusing on one goal.

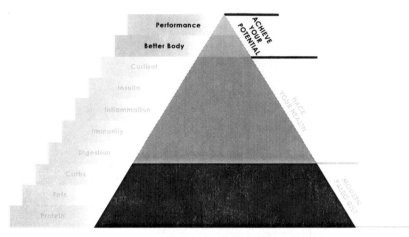

Figure D. The Paleo Project Pyramid—Section III

Being able to deadlift 400lb doesn't necessarily make you leaner or give you six-pack abs. On the other hand, competing as a high-level hockey player at 6% body fat doesn't necessarily make you a better player than you would be at 10% body fat. The clearer your goals, the better you can implement the *correct* strategy and achieve the *best* results! Once you have achieved your primary goal, you can then shift your focus and tackle the other goal if you choose to.

Not sure what your primary goal should be? Have a look at the following scenarios and see if there is one that best fits your current situation.

"I feel that if I could just trim 5-10lb, I would be able to run a faster marathon."

In this case, your ultimate goal is *to complete a faster time*, to perform better. By completing the steps in Chapter 10 and focusing on performance you will likely also lose weight. You will prioritize the training regimen that will support improved performance while not adversely affecting your lean muscle, strength and power. If you were trying to lose weight, you could jeopardize your performance by simply trying to reduce the number on the scale.

"My doctor has told me that I need to lose weight and exercise because I have high blood pressure."

In this scenario, your goal is *better body composition* and ultimately better health. By completing the steps in Chapter 9, you will learn the exercise and movement strategy best suited to improving your health, including your blood pressure. The program will also detail the best dietary strategy and cardio regimen to achieve your goals.

"My coaches have told me that I really need to add 8-10 pounds of muscle in order to compete at the next level."

For this athlete, the primary goal is *adding muscle mass*, therefore *performance* is the goal. In Chapter 10, I'll outline the dietary strategy necessary to increase your lean muscle mass. When your goal is to increase size, you shouldn't be overly concerned with a nominal increase in body fat. To get bigger and add lean muscle, you need the proper hormonal terrain and surplus of calories to support your goals.

"I want to look better AND perform better at work."

This is a very common refrain in clinical practice. By working your way through the plan in Chapter 9, will achieve rapid fat loss, look better, and as a result you'll see improvements in many others areas of the body (blood sugar and insulin control, cortisol stress balance, and cognitive function.) Once you've achieved your best body, you could then proceed to Chapter 10. However, for some, Chapter 9 will be the end of the road because they will have realized all the goals on their journey.

Determining your primary goal, whether it's fat loss/body composition or performance, will influence how you fuel your body (ratio of protein, carbohydrates and fats), what you consume around bouts of training, and what the type of exercise you perform. The quickest path between two points is a straight line and that is the path you will take if you define the direction you want to take.

Over the next eight weeks, follow the roadmap I lay out in *either* Chapter 9 or 10 to help you build your best body or achieve a new personal best. In Chapter 9, I'll describe the key hormones that influence your quest for weight loss and better health. I'll dispel common fat loss myths and then provide you with my *Better Body Plan* for success.

In Chapter 10, I'll discuss the key anabolic hormones that are crucial for increasing lean mass and upgrading your performance, as well as my top five performance principles. Then I will outline my *Performance Plan*, a detailed diet, exercise and supplement regimen to maximize your progress and achieve your performance potential.

You've done all the hard work up to this point; now you are ready to push to the finish line!

CHAPTER 9

UPGRADE YOUR BODY—The Better Body Plan

One of the most common reasons it's so difficult to maintain your ideal body is because the world around you is overweight and out of shape. Can you believe that 75% of the population of North America is classified as overweight or obese? Our current lifestyle (always "on the run"), food supply (laden with processed foods, hidden sugars and GMO foods) and level of activity (or inactivity) conspire together to lead us down the weight gain path. Unfortunately, if you simply go with the flow, you'll likely end up downstream in the same boat—overweight, tired and unhealthy!

In *Section I,* you learned how to build the foundation for the best diet in the world—the Modern Paleo diet—optimizing your intake of quality proteins, healthy fats, nutrient rich veggies, fruit, and gluten-free carbs. In *Section II,* you hacked your health to uncover areas of imbalance or deficiency and subsequently upgraded your digestion, immunity, inflammation control and hormone balance. Now, you are primed and ready to lose weight, upgrade your health and build a better body.

The late, great Jack Lalanne was considered the "godfather of fitness." He was renowned for his incredible feats like swimming *handcuffed* from Alcatraz to Fisherman's Wharf in San Francisco and setting the world record for push-ups with 1,033 in 23 minutes! Jack was a pioneer of fitness and nutrition and his mantra for fat loss was straightforward: "The best way to get fat off is to eat less and exercise more!" This may sound harsh, but its simplicity is its success—*if* you know exactly *how* you should be eating and *how* you should be exercising.

In order to right the ship and achieve your *best body,* I've outlined in this chapter the most efficient diet, exercise and supplement plan for you to trigger fast and long-term fat loss. Before you get started, I discuss key hormones that influence fat loss, some common fat loss myths and where people typically go wrong.

I. KEY HORMONES FOR FAT LOSS

Insulin Sensitivity and Fat-burning Potential

In Chapter 7, I outlined the importance of managing insulin levels in order to improve your health and support weight loss. Remember that *insulin sensitivity* is a measure of how efficiently your body is able to process carbohydrates. As a general rule, the leaner or fitter you are, the better your insulin sensitivity.

On the other hand, the more overweight or out of shape you are, the more insulin *insensitive* you become. This means that your insulin receptors are no longer as efficient at getting glucose into cells, requiring your body to produce more and more insulin to do the job.

The problem with the typical Western diet is that it's too high in carbohydrates and simple sugars, particularly at breakfast time. High glycemic carbs and sugary treats elevate your insulin and blood sugar levels, shown in Figure 9.1, reducing cAMP levels and turning off your fat-burning potential (HSL). It's not a great way to start the day if you are trying to lose weight!

Chronically high blood insulin levels will predispose you to poor insulin sensitivity and ultimately insulin resistance, leaving you stuck in fat-building mode. Insulin resistance is a hallmark of chronic weight gain and poor health and, if you continue down this road, a greater risk of developing type-II diabetes. If you successfully made it through the

Insulin Action Plan in Chapter 7 then you are already on your way to restoring optimal insulin function.

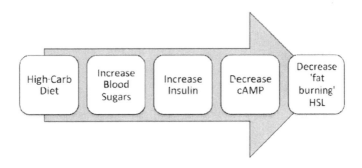

Figure 9.1. Insulin Inhibits Fat-Burning HSL

The Thyroid Gland and Your Metabolic Rate

Located on the anterior surface of your throat, your thyroid gland is responsible for setting your metabolic rate by producing hormones that determine how fast (or slowly) your metabolic engine runs. It's your body's thermostat, controlling how much energy you burn to maintain normal physiologic functions (i.e., keep you alive).

If you are overweight or have steadily gained weight over the years you may have a sluggish thyroid—the term used to describe a *slowing* of your metabolic rate. The slower your metabolism, the more likely you are to gain weight.

If you have a sluggish thyroid, your brain produces increasing amounts of thyroid stimulating hormone (TSH) from the pituitary gland, which tells your thyroid gland to work harder! The thyroid gland responds to this request by increasing the production of the thyroid hormone *thyroxine* (also called T4). The T4 hormone travels through your bloodstream to tell the rest of your body to get moving and increase metabolism.

In order to complete its task, T4 must be converted into its active form *triiodothyronine (T3)* inside your cells. The hormone T3 is directly responsible for metabolic rate, growth and development and is dependent on the presence of selenium to convert T4 into the active T3. Low selenium levels mean low conversion rates and subsequently slower metabolism. If you are already on thyroid medications, it's important to note they act only to increase T4 and not the active T3. If you are deficient in selenium, you will be much more susceptible to sub-optimal thyroid function.

Stress and Sluggish Thyroid Function

One of the primary reasons for sluggish thyroid function is stress. In Chapter 8, I described how hectic work and home schedules, as well as an intense exercise regimen increase stress (cortisol and adrenaline) levels and tax your adrenal glands.

When your adrenal glands are working overtime, your thyroid gland attempts to pick up some of the workload and help out. While this attempt to increase your metabolic rate will help you keep your energy up in the short term, in the long term it can wear out your thyroid gland.

Elevated TSH levels are commonly seen when the adrenals are taxed, leading to sluggish thyroid function, slower metabolism and subsequent weight gain. The normal lab values for TSH range from 0.35-5.00. Ideally, your TSH levels should be less than 2.0. If your lab results show levels greater than 2.0 and you are overweight, you may have early signs of a sluggish thyroid. This is referred to as a *functional deficiency*— you exhibit the signs and symptoms of hypothyroidism without your TSH levels being outside the normal range.

If this scenario persists for long enough, you may develop low thyroid function and be diagnosed with a hypothyroid condition. Hypothyroidism is five times more common in women. Symptoms include fatigue, cold intolerance, depression, weight gain, weakness, joint aches, constipation, dry skin, hair loss and menstrual irregularities.[1] Rather than waiting until your values get outside the normal range, start supporting your thyroid (and adrenals) with the right mix of diet and exercise in order to restore balance.

Estrogen and Weight Gain

Estrogen is the dominant hormone in women, increasing in the first two weeks after menstruation to stimulate the build-up of tissue in the uterus and the development of eggs in the ovaries. It is produced primarily in the ovaries but also by your adrenal glands and body fat tissue. This is an important point because if you are overweight, your fat cells will ramp up the production of estrogen, further exacerbating the weight-gain cycle.

Few men realize they also need estrogen to promote optimal health, although in smaller quantities compared to women. Estrogen is important for cardiovascular health, balancing blood sugars, increasing good HDL cholesterol and supporting deep sleep.

The problem starts when men gain too much body fat, because testosterone gets rapidly converted to estrogen via increases in the *aromatase* enzyme (this can also occur in women). If you have a beer belly or fat accumulation around the chest, you are especially vulnerable to increased aromatase activity.

Women with elevated body-fat levels or a shapely hourglass figure tend to have higher estrogen levels. Other common causes of high estrogen levels or *estrogen dominance* are xeno-estrogens (present in herbicides, pesticides and plastics), stress, poor liver function (high alcohol intake) and constipation. A urine test can be performed to measure an estrogen metabolite (16-alpha-hydrozyestrone) that is associated with estrogen dominance.

In both men and women, a combination of elevated estrogen and insulin levels, along with a sluggish thyroid, are the perfect storm for weight gain!

II. FAT LOSS MYTHS BUSTED!

1) A Calorie is *Not* Just a Calorie

You've probably always been told that the key to weight loss is to simply reduce your calories. Nutritionists, dieticians and doctors have passed on the belief that a calorie is a calorie, a form of nutritional accounting that has little regard for whether the calories were consumed by eating an apple pie or avocados.

Proponents of calorie counting base their argument on the scientific laws of thermodynamics to support their view of nutritional accounting. Unfortunately, this theory is not consistent with the actual laws of thermodynamics. (I think they must have missed a few physics classes!) Let me review.

Newton's first law of thermodynamics states that energy is neither created nor destroyed, thus implying to classical nutritionists that all calories affect the body in exactly the same way. Unfortunately, this ignores Newton's second law of thermodynamics, which states that in any irreversible reaction (e.g., eating food), entropy must always increase. This is a fancy way of saying that balance of energy (i.e., calories) is not expected![2] Strike one against counting calories.

The nutritional accounting strategy also fails to take into account how the food you are eating affects your hormones. For example, one person eats a high protein breakfast (six eggs at 144 calories), while the other has a small bowl of corn flakes (also 144 calories). Compare the effects of each of these meals on the body.

The high protein breakfast increases glucagon levels—an important trigger for fat loss—as well as your dopamine levels, which are the feel-good neurotransmitters that make you focused, alert and ready for the day. In addition, protein raises your *thermic effect of food* (TEF), meaning you will burn more energy by eating protein versus carbs.

In contrast, the high-carb meal dramatically increases your blood sugar and insulin levels, thereby reducing your fat-burning potential. This typically leads to blood sugar swings throughout the day and cravings for sugar. Strike two against calorie counting.

Finally, did you know that the calorie content listed on food labels can be wrong by as much as a whopping 30% or more! Harvard scientist Richard Wrangham notes in his research that while *processed food* calorie counts are pretty accurate, *whole foods* often have far *fewer* calories than listed. Also, calorie counts for healthy foods ignore the energy required to digest and assimilate the food, misleading consumers into thinking that processed foods are the healthier option. Strike three to calorie counting! To summarize, stop wasting your time counting calories. At the end of this chapter, I show you how to shift your consumption so that you can put your calculator away forever!

2) Multiple Meals (4-6) Are *Not* Always Best For Fat Loss

Eating meals every three to four hours is a common suggestion made by nutritionists and personal trainers to improve body composition. The reasoning is that increased meal frequency helps to stabilize blood sugar and insulin levels, increasing your metabolism and ability to burn fat. This strategy is proven to help some people but it's not the whole story.

A study in the *British Journal of Nutrition* (2010) compared people eating three meals a day versus those consuming three meals + three snacks daily. After eight weeks, the results showed no difference in body fat and appetite measurements.[3] Ultimately, eating multiple meals might be holding you back from achieving your weight loss goals.

How many meals should you eat per day? A recent Dutch study compared the difference between high meal frequency versus low meal frequency on metabolism. The results showed that something very interesting happened to the low meal frequency group. The group eating just three square meals a day exhibited greater appetite control, superior blood sugar control and increased resting metabolic rate![4] The group eating three meals per day had fewer cravings, more consistent energy and a faster metabolism. Pretty impressive!

If three meals per day will accelerate your fat loss then you may be thinking why not bump it down to two meals? Well, it seems less is not always better. If you decrease your meals from three to two per day, you decrease your satiety levels and ability to burn fat.[5] Therefore, stick with three meals per day for best results. ***Note:*** This does not mean

EVERYONE should only eat three meals a day, but if your weight loss is stagnant and you are a regular snacker during the day, it may be the catalyst to get you back on the right track.

On the other hand, a study in the journal *Obesity* (2013) compared the impact of consuming three high protein meals per day versus six high-protein meals per day on weight loss in overweight subjects. The results showed that six high protein meals per day resulted in decreased body fat and abdominal fat, increased lean body mass and accelerated caloric after-burn post training.[6] This may sound confusing—both three meals a day and six meals per day are best for promoting fat loss?

So, which is best? Essentially, inducing *hormesis* (positive adaptations) results from *changing* what you are currently doing. This means if you want to maximize weight loss, you'll get the best results by *eating differently* from your norm. I outline the program in more detail at the end of this chapter.

DIET DIARIES—MEN ARE FROM MARS AND WOMEN ARE FROM VENUS

When it comes to weight loss and diet diaries, it seems that men and women are quite different. A new study examined the impact of using diet diaries versus online forums in an attempt to find the best way to improve weight loss.

Interestingly, the use of a diet diary predicted a significant reduction in weight for men, but not for women![7] When men were asked to note down all the foods they consumed on a daily basis, it resulted in better eating habits and superior results.

Diet diaries did not improve outcomes for women, but they did show excellent progress with the use of online chat forums. It seems women have more success when they were able to share their experiences and hear about the successes and struggles of others. Being a part of the online community predicted a significant loss of weight in women, but not in men!

These results show the differences between men and women when it comes to strategies to support the weight loss process.

3) Endurance Training is *Not* The Best For Fat Loss

Continuous cardiovascular exercise is classically viewed as the best way to burn fat. It works by increasing calcium levels in your muscle tissue, which leads to the production of *PGC-1 alpha*, your fat-burning master switch. When PGC-1 alpha is activated, a series of positive metabolic adaptations occur that improve your insulin sensitivity, increase the number of mitochondria and therefore improve your ability to burn fat.

However, cardio is no longer the fat-burning king. Over the past decade, new research on shorter, more intense bouts of aerobic exercise (called high-intensity interval training or HIIT) has turned the cardio for fat-loss theory completely upside down. Researchers discovered that HIIT activates PGC-1 alpha—your fat burning master switch—via a completely different pathway. This means that HIIT can produce *even greater benefits* than endurance training *in far less time*!

Not convinced? Take a closer look at the research and see how endurance training stack ups head to head against HIIT training for fat loss.

Excess Post-exercise Oxygen Consumption (EPOC)

Excess post-exercise oxygen consumption (EPOC) is a fancy way of saying the "after burn" your body experiences after a hard workout. It is the amount of oxygen required by your body to offset the oxygen shortage that occurred during your training. It sounds pretty complicated, but essentially EPOC is the calories you burn once your exercise is over.

After you finish your workout, you continue to burn calories because oxygen is required to bring your body back to a state of equilibrium. The harder your interval training is, the greater your EPOC. The greater your EPOC, the more calories you'll burn sitting at your desk or in your car after your workout.[8] (A major reason why weight training, CrossFit, and sprint training are all fantastic for losing weight and getting leaner!)

Fat Burning

HIIT achieves *greater fat burning* than steady state endurance training. The rise in EPOC after HIIT triggers the breakdown of body fat, which is used as fuel during your recovery phase. This massive post-exercise effect is actually greater than the amount of fat you would have burned doing an hour on the treadmill at a steady pace. That's right—you will burn more calories standing in line waiting for your lunch after a HIIT session than you would logging all those miles on the treadmill!

VO2 Max

Maximal oxygen consumption or VO2 max is the gold standard for measuring your aerobic horsepower and is defined as the body's maximum capacity for transporting and using oxygen during intense exercise. Traditionally, building an aerobic base has been the hallmark for generating a higher V02 max. However, the latest research shows that HIIT training is superior to aerobic training in developing a higher VO2 max.[8] This is a tremendous advantage for weight loss clients, as well as anyone trying to improve their fitness!

Cardiac Parameters

Endurance training is good for your heart, improving many important cardiovascular parameters vital for performance and overall health, including stroke volume, cardiac contractility and cardiac hypertrophy. Traditionally, endurance training has been thought to be the best method of improving these parameters. Did you know that HIIT shows equal ability to improve cardiac markers compared to aerobic training? In essence, it's a tie on this one. Check out the summary of how HIIT training stacks up against traditional cardio in Figure 9.2.

If you want to lose weight, improve your energy and overall health, start incorporating HIIT into your routine today. Unless you are training for a specific endurance competition, skip the long steady sessions and get more efficient with your training.

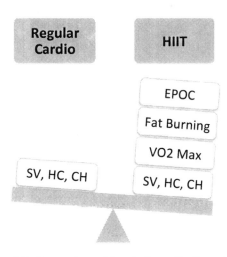

Figure 9.2. Comparison of Steady-State Cardio vs. HIIT

III. THE BETTER BODY PLAN

THE 3-STEP PLAN

1. Testing—Set Your Baseline

2. Keto-Paleo Diet—The Best Fat Loss Diet in the World

3. Exercise—The Most Efficient Fat Loss Program

STEP 1. TESTING
Know Your Body Composition
Getting your body composition tested is essential when starting any fat loss protocol. You must establish your *starting point* before you can set your destination. Baseline measurements are crucial for tracking progress and identifying any roadblocks on your journey to a better body. Not having baseline tests is like driving without a roadmap. It means you are destined to take the scenic route!

Caliper Testing
Skinfold caliper testing should be your first choice for measuring your body composition—your levels of lean muscle and body fat. Caliper testing measures the thickness of your skinfolds at various points on your body by pinching subcutaneous fat. These measurements are then inserted into a mathematical formula to calculate your lean muscle mass, fat mass and body-fat percentage. The caliper testing provides the practitioner with valuable information regarding the type of fat you are predominantly storing (bad white fat versus good brown fat) and the specific areas you are storing fat. For example, the abdominal skinfold site is associated with fluctuations in cortisol stress levels.

Be sure to find a qualified professional to perform your test because becoming proficient in caliper testing takes several years of experience. Inaccuracies occur most commonly from poor technique in novice testers.[9]

Tape Measurements
Tape measurements are useful in evaluating changes in body composition. They are easy to perform and provide you with additional data for measuring your progress. For general health, waist circumference should be less than 38 inches (102cm) in men and 36 inches (88cm) in women. Waist circumference is a powerful indicator of increased risk of chronic diseases such as high blood pressure, high cholesterol, heart disease, diabetes and cancer.[10]

THE SCALE IS NOT YOUR FRIEND

If you are only using a scale at home to track your weight-loss progress, your success will be doomed! Why? Your body is made up of approximately two-thirds water, which means dehydration is the quickest way to lose weight. Unfortunately, this is the secret behind most fad diets or supplement pills.

Another reason your scale is not a good measure of success is that lean muscle weighs a lot more than fat. Think of muscle as bricks and fat as beach balls. If you lose muscle your weight will drop, but so too will your metabolic rate—not a good recipe for long-term success.

When you lose muscle on fad diets and detox regimes, you lose precious muscle glycogen stores. For every molecule of glycogen in your muscles, you carry three molecules of water. Losing muscle tissue translates into reduced glycogen stores, resulting in further weight loss but not fat loss (another trick of gimmicky fad diets!).

Losing muscle, glycogen and water is not the kind of weight loss you are after. It's fool's gold that inevitably leads to high cortisol stress levels, insulin imbalance, a sluggish metabolism and of course weight gain. Save yourself from this mess and lose weight the right way.

STEP 2. THE <u>BEST</u> FAT LOSS DIET IN THE WORLD
THE KETOGENIC DIET

Magazines, newspaper and fad diet books are filled with trendy and exotic diets, all claiming to be the next "miracle cure" for weight loss. While these may seem to be your ticket to fat loss, you'll likely be disappointed in the long run.

The truth is, you don't need a fad diet. The science behind which diet is best for fat loss is quite clear—the ketogenic diet is head and shoulders above the rest.

A *ketogenic diet* is the scientific term for a *very* low-carb diet (50g of carbs daily, whereas a *low-carb* diet is approximately 100g daily), named after the ketone compounds produced by the body when carbohydrate intake is reduced. The benefits of lowering your total carbohydrate intake and adopting a *ketogenic* or *low-carbohydrate diet,* shown in Figure 9.3, include: improving insulin balance, increasing satiety, cooling inflammation and losing weight.[11] Kick-start your metabolism and drop a dress size or pant size in no time!

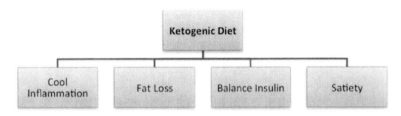

Figure 9.3. Benefits of a Ketogenic Diet

Balances Insulin

If improving insulin balance is a key factor in successful long-term weight loss, it makes sense to modify the macronutrient that most directly affects insulin output—carbohydrates! A ketogenic diet is a powerful tool for correcting dysfunctional insulin levels in the body.

Clinical studies confirm the ketogenic diet improves insulin resistance, a hallmark of long-term weight loss and poor health.[12, 13]

Burns More Fat, Increases Satiety

The metabolic transformation on a ketogenic diet happens very quickly, over the course of several weeks, as your body shifts from using carbs as its primary fuel source to fats.

Recently, a study compared the effects of *low-carb* diets versus *low-fat* diets on fat loss over a three to six month period. The results were impressive. The very low-carb group lost *twice* as much weight as the low-fat group.[14] This wasn't the only benefit of low-carb eating for fat loss. The low-carb group said they felt greater satiety throughout the day, which researchers attributed to the *7x greater ketone levels* in those on the ketogenic diet.

The ketones act as an appetite suppressant, making you feel full for longer periods through the day instead of craving your next sugar fix. In fact, a growing body of evidence is showing that ketones may in fact be *super fuels,* up to 25% more efficient at producing ATP (your body's primary energy currency) than the standard glucose or fatty acids (now that is a complete 180 degree shift in thinking!).[12]

Reduces Inflammation

In Chapter 6, I discussed how weight gain results in chronically elevated inflammatory levels. Increased abdominal circumference is a reliable marker of inflammation, accumulation of visceral fat and poor general health. As the fires of inflammation burn hotter, it worsens the weight-gain cycle.

How can you reverse this process? Adopting a ketogenic diet will help cool excess inflammation and reduce harmful free radical damage. Studies show an *approximately 50% reduction* in key inflammatory markers (CRP, TNF, IL-6).[13,14] Ultimately, this will set you up for long-term sustainable weight loss.

THE "KETO-PALEO" DIET

In Section I, I described the platform for the healthiest diet in the world—the Modern Paleo diet. Now, you will take that foundation and transform it into the perfect weight loss plan. The protocol is simple: blend the Paleo diet with a ketogenic approach and you have the world's best weight loss diet. The Paleo diet's emphasis on quality proteins, healthy fats and an abundant intake of vegetables make it the perfect pairing for a ketogenic weight-loss diet.

Be sure to adhere to the principles laid out in Section I and include a daily intake of the following:

• Protein – eat 1.5-2.0g/kg of your bodyweight daily

- Fat – at least 1.5-2.0 thumb-sized portions per meal for men; at least 1.0-1.5 thumbs per meal for women

- Leafy greens – as many as you want!

- Cruciferous veggies – as many as you want! (cooked)

- Fruit – minimal (fruit juice NOT allowed)

- Complex carbs – minimal to none

Listed below is a sample "Keto-Paleo" diet for the Phase I and II *Better Body Plan*.

SAMPLE KETO-PALEO DIET: MEN

PHASE I (WEEKS 1-4), THREE MEALS PER DAY

Breakfast
Protein shake (40g) + ½ *large* avocado + handful spinach + blueberries (½ cup)

Lunch
Haddock + sautéed kale (1 cup) + cherry tomatoes (½ cup) + orange bell pepper (1 medium) + olive oil (2tbsp extra-virgin)

Dinner
Turkey breast (one and a half) + steamed broccoli + butter/ghee (2 tbsp) + dessert 1/2 cup (frozen grapes)

	Proteins (g)	Fats (g)	Carbs (g)
Breakfast	45	15	20
Lunch	44	30	20
Dinner	46	30	15
	135	75	55

PHASE II (WEEKS 5-8), FIVE MEALS PER DAY

Breakfast
Eggs (x 4) + bacon (2 slices) + cherry tomatoes (1 cup)

Snack AM
Greek yogurt (150g non-fat) + walnuts (x 7 halves) + green tea

Lunch
Grass-fed beef (6oz rib eye) + stir-fry collard greens (1 cup) + olive oil (1 tbsp extra-virgin)

Snack PM
Whey isolate protein shake (40g) + coconut oil (1 tbsp) + water

Dinner

Wild salmon (½ fillet) + roasted Brussels sprouts (1 cup) + butter/ghee (1 tbsp) + dessert (½ cup pineapple)

	Proteins (g)	Fats (g)	Carbs (g)
Breakfast	31	23.5	10
Snack AM	13	13	2
Lunch	43	20	12
Snack PM	40	15	0
Dinner	44	28	22
	171	99.5	46

SAMPLE KETO-PALEO DIET: FEMALE

PHASE I (WEEKS 1-4), THREE MEALS PER DAY

Breakfast

Protein shake (30g) + ½ *large* avocado + handful spinach + blueberries (½ cup)

Lunch

Haddock + sautéed kale (1 cup) + cherry tomatoes (½ cup) + orange bell pepper (1 medium) + olive oil (1 tbsp extra-virgin)

Dinner

Turkey breast (x1) + steamed broccoli + butter/ghee (1 tbsp) + dessert (1/2 cup frozen grapes)

	Proteins (g)	Fats (g)	Carbs (g)
Breakfast	35	10.5	20
Lunch	44.5	14.5	20
Dinner	32.5	15	15
	112	40	55

Breakfast

Eggs (x 3) + bacon (1 slice) + cherry tomatoes (1 cup)

Snack AM

Greek yogurt (100g non-fat) + walnuts (7 halves) + green tea

Lunch

Grass-fed beef (4oz rib eye) + stir-fry collard greens (1 cup) + olive oil (½ cup extra-virgin)

Snack PM

Whey isolate protein shake (30g) + coconut oil (½ tbsp) + water

Dinner

Wild salmon (½ fillet) + roasted Brussels sprouts (1 cup) + butter/ghee (½ tbsp) + dessert (½ cup pineapple)

	Proteins (g)	Fats (g)	Carbs (g)
Breakfast	22	21	11
Snack AM	9	9	2
Lunch	30	8	11
Snack PM	30	7.5	0
Dinner	44	21	22
	135	66.5	46

INTERMITTENT FASTING FOR FAT LOSS

Intermittent Fasting (IF) is a new spin on weight loss based on altering your meal frequency to accelerate fat loss. It involves fasting for 16 straight hours of the day and feasting during the remaining eight hours.

How does it work? Simply delay your breakfast until 10 a.m., follow that with lunch at 2 p.m., and then finish with dinner at 6 p.m. That is your eight straight hours of eating. If these times don't work for you, simply push back your first meal to noon and you can have dinner at 8 p.m.

After dinner, you'll have a 16-hour fasting period before your next day's breakfast. When you take into account seven to eight hours of sleep per night, it's not as difficult as you might think.

The theory behind intermittent fasting is that after a night's sleep you wake up in the perfect hormonal terrain for fat burning—low insulin and high glucagon levels that trigger the breakdown of fat. IF can be a great recipe for fat loss but it must be used appropriately.

FACTORS TO CONSIDER

There are no miracle fat-loss cures. Intermittent fasting can be effective but it must be used in the right scenario to get the desired results. It's not for everyone. The following three factors must be in good order before you start your IF program:

- You must already be eating a healthy, well-rounded diet.
- You must have no trouble falling asleep or staying asleep at night.
- You must have a normal cortisol rhythm. If you are very busy or stressed, IF can worsen your cortisol response.

If any of these factors are out of balance, starting an IF protocol is a bad idea because it can exacerbate cortisol dysfunction and lead to dramatic energy swings, depressed mood and possible weight gain (not loss!).

Interestingly, men tend to achieve superior results with IF than women. Female hormones are more complex and more negative side effects are seen in women using long-term IF than in men.

STEP 3. THE <u>BEST</u> EXERCISE PLAN—FAT LOSS AND BODY COMPOSITION

Diet and exercise are the foundation of any good weight-loss program. Exercise is a powerful weapon for improving insulin sensitivity and setting yourself up for long-term weight-loss success. The key is to be efficient with your time and train the right way, incorporating a combination of weight training and cardio (HIIT) to accelerate your progress.

"HIIT" CARDIO TRAINING

When was the last time you ran as fast as you could? For many people, you might have to go all the way back to high school or even grade school! There are tremendous benefits to exerting yourself to your fullest (no matter how far or how fast you are going). High intensity interval training (HIIT) is your secret weapon to achieving your best body in the quickest time possible.

My two favourite methods are sprints (outdoors, no treadmills) or the stationary bike in your gym. A major benefit of sprinting is that it reduces the amount of ground contact time compared to jogging for long periods of time. This translates to less pounding on your joints. If you are new to running or sprinting, simply start slowly and build up your speed gradually over several weeks or months.

Beginner HIIT Protocol

To start, find a nearby track or simply pace off the desired distance in your local park or on a quiet street. At the outset of each session, warm up gently for three to five minutes with a light jog and then sprint!

Here is your plan for the next eight weeks. Perform each workout *twice* weekly:

Phase I

WEEK	WORKOUT (Sets × Distance)	REST PERIOD
1	6 × 50m	60s
2	7 × 50m	60s
3	8 × 50m	60s
4	10 × 50m	60s

Phase II

WEEK	WORKOUT (Sets × Distance)	REST PERIOD
5	6 × 100m	60s
6	7 × 100m	60s
7	8 × 100m	60s
8	10 × 100m	60s

Moderate/Advanced HIIT Protocol

Here is your plan for the next eight weeks. Perform each workout *three* times weekly:

Phase I

WEEK	WORKOUT (Sets × Distance)	REST PERIOD
1	8 × 50m	60s
2	10 × 50m	60s
3	12 × 50m	60s
4	15 × 50m	60s

Phase II

WEEK	WORKOUT (Sets × Distance)	REST PERIOD
5	8 × 100m	60s
6	10 × 100m	60s
7	12 × 100m	60s
8	15 × 100m	60s

STRENGTH TRAINING

Strength training triggers an overwhelming number of positive adaptations that promote fat loss and superior overall health, such as improving insulin and blood sugars, boosting testosterone levels, increasing metabolic rate, reducing cortisol stress response, decreasing inflammation, normalizing gut health, improving liver function and the list goes on! There is no drug or food in the world that can produce so many positive changes in your body as weight training.

If you are new to training the best part is you don't have to lift heavy weights. During your training sessions, your focus should be on maximizing the *time under tension* (TUT)—your total work time—because this produces superior energy expenditure, regardless of the number of repetitions.[16] Stop counting all those reps. Just put on some great music, set a timer on your phone for 60 second-intervals per exercise and away you go!

Not sure where to start? Complete the *Strength Training For Fat Loss & Body Composition* routine listed in *Appendix C* to accelerate your progress and achieve your best body. The program involves training two to three days per week over the next eight weeks.

If you're experienced in the gym then weight training is probably already part of your regimen. Therefore, if you are *still* struggling to lose weight, you need to re-assess your exercise selection, repetitions, rest periods and periodization to ensure it's designed to meet your fat-loss goals. Frequently, I find clients go wrong by not including enough *intensity* and *density* in their training. What does this mean?

Intensity is quite straightforward. It's how hard you are working. Typically, when clients struggle with weight loss they add *more volume* (not intensity) to their training, meaning more training days during the week. However, if you want better results the research is very clear—you need to focus on increasing exercise *intensity* (how hard you train). This doesn't mean lifting the heaviest possible weight, but rather working to exhaustion (when you are unable to perform repetitions with perfect form).

Training density is when you aim to perform more work in the same allotted time during your training sessions. The more reps and sets you can perform in that time, the greater your *training density*. This dramatically increases your ability to burn fat and improves your body composition. In my opinion, one of the best methods of increasing your training density is CrossFit or CrossFit-style training. Try adding two sessions per week over four weeks.

Finally, incorporating more Energy Systems work—sled pulls, farmer's walks, prowler pushes, sprints—at the end of training sessions (or on cardio days) may provide the boost you need to get leaner. If you have tried everything and nothing seems to work then some comprehensive lab testing may uncover systems imbalances described in Section II.

SUMMARY OF EXERCISE PLAN

Let me review a sample week of your Better Body Exercise Plan:

BEGINNER – PHASE I – First 4 Weeks (1-4)

Monday	Tuesday	Wednesday	Thursday	Friday	Saturday	Sunday
Weights or CrossFit	Sprints	Rest or yoga	Weights or CrossFit	Sprints	Rest or yoga	Long walk

BEGINNER – PHASE II – Next 4 Weeks (5-8)

Monday	Tuesday	Wednesday	Thursday	Friday	Saturday	Sunday
Weights or CrossFit	Sprints	Weights	Sprints	Rest or yoga	Weights or CrossFit	Long walk

(Increase weight training to three sessions per week)

MODERATE/ADVANCED – PHASE I - First 4 Weeks (1-4)

Monday	Tuesday	Wednesday	Thursday	Friday	Saturday	Sunday
CrossFit or Metabolic Conditioning	Sprints	Weights	Sprints	CrossFit or Metabolic Conditioning	Sprints	Rest or gentle yoga

MODERATE/ADVANCED – PHASE II - Next 4 Weeks (5-8)

Monday	Tuesday	Wednesday	Thursday	Friday	Saturday	Sunday
CrossFit or Metabolic Conditioning	Weight training PM: Sprints	Yoga	CrossFit or Metabolic Conditioning	AM: Weight training PM: Sprints	Sprints or yoga	Rest

(Increase weight training to four sessions per week, add sprints post-training two sessions per week and add one yoga session per week)

DO I NEED TO SUPPLEMENT?

If you are struggling to lose weight or to see changes in your body composition through diet and exercise, it's time to consider adding supplementation. Start by adding the Insulin Action Plan described in Chapter 7 (all three levels), for 12 weeks.

1. Cinnamon

2. Alpha-Lipoic Acid (ALA)

3. Berberine

Be sure to get the appropriate lab tests done before embarking on any supplement protocol, so you can track your progress.

As for fat-burning supplements—save your money! In fact, would you believe the best supplement for promoting fat loss is probably already in your kitchen? That's right—the caffeine from your coffee is pound for pound the best thermogenic or fat-burner on the market! (It's also the secret ingredient in virtually all fat burning products!).

Before you add coffee to your routine, your adrenals have to be in good working order (i.e., you scored PASS on your Adrenal self-assessment in Chapter 8. If not, stick with drinking green tea). If so, try adding a cup of coffee before your morning training sessions to accelerate fat burning and improve your work capacity. Remember, stick to one coffee per day and always before noon.

CASE STUDY—WEIGHT LOSS

Tracy, a 34-year-old lawyer, came to me wanting to lose weight and regain the physique she had five years prior. She had gained weight slowly over the past five years as the demands from her career increased. She no longer went to the gym, she ate most of her meals at the office and her weekend leisure activities were now fewer and further between.

Tracy weighed 165lb (5'7 tall) and wanted to drop 15 pounds, lose her self-described "muffin top" and generally feel healthier. She relied heavily on caffeine and sweet snacks throughout the day to keep her energy levels up. Tracy had no problem falling asleep, but struggled to sleep through the night and woke up in the morning very tired. Her meals were always eaten on the go, a mix of fast food, restaurants and her office cafeteria. She admitted to having chronic bloating and abdominal discomfort.

Her lab tests, shown in Figure 9.4, revealed the following:

Lab Test	Normal Range	Tracy's Levels	Significance
CRP-hs	Optimal less than 1.0	2.6	High normal – Sign of low level systemic inflammation
Fasting Insulin	Optimal less than 50	98	High normal – Early sign of insulin insensitivity
HA1c	Optimal less than 0.55	0.59	High normal – Sign of mildly elevated blood sugars over past 3 months
Fructoseamine	Optimal less than 180	270	High normal - Sign of mildly elevated blood sugars over past 3 weeks
Triglycerides	Optimal less than 1.00	1.8	High normal – Associated with poor insulin sensitivity
GGT	Less than 30	44	High – Associated with poor diet or high alcohol consumption
Secretory IgA (stool)	50-200	268	High – Possible leaky gut and food allergies
Bacterial Culture (stool)	*Expected Flora* Bifidobacterium spp. +3-4 Lactobacillus spp. +3-4	*Expected Flora* Bifidobacterium spp. +NG Lactobacillus spp. +1	Insufficient 'good' gut bacteria.
	Dysbiotic Flora None present	*Dysbiotic Flora* Gamma hemo. strep +3 Alpha hemo. strep +3 Enterobacter aerog. +3 Candida albicans +2	Presence of dysbiotic 'bad' gut bacteria & yeasts

Figure 9.4. Summary of Tracy's Initial Lab Test Results

Tracy had to make some major changes in her diet and lifestyle to meet her goals. Fortunately, she was motivated to get started and had the resources to enlist a food service for her three meals. I put her on a very low-carb keto-Paleo diet for eight weeks, eliminated coffee completely (replacing it with green tea) and removed all sugars from her diet. Her only other food was a whey protein shake in the afternoon before training.

The dietary changes would help lay the foundation for improving Tracy's gut health, but she needed more support in the short term. Therefore, I added anti-microbial berberine to eliminated dysbiotic bacteria, a probiotic supplement twice daily to support gut flora and a blend of glutamine, zinc and quercetin at bedtime to correct her leaky gut.

Finally, she agreed she could carve out four 30-minute sessions per week and hired a trainer twice weekly to walk her through the weight-training routine, while performing the HIIT training on her own.

Tracy emailed me after one week and confessed she felt more tired, lethargic and struggled with headaches and irritability (very common symptoms when caffeine is removed from the diet). I told her this was a normal reaction to making all the changes and that she should stay the course. She was not thrilled but decided to stick with it.

I was pleased to receive her email after Week 2. Her energy levels were improving, she was sleeping more soundly through the night, and she had dropped five pounds. At our four-week follow-up, she looked far more energetic. The bags under her eyes were clearing, she was more vibrant and engaging and she said her digestive distress (constant gas and bloating) were now completely gone. She had lost 10 pounds (8 pounds fat mass) and was looking and feeling much better.

Finally, after 12 weeks, Tracy came back into my office and apologized for her stern email after Week 1 (I didn't think it was that bad!). She couldn't remember the last time her energy levels were this good, when she could sleep through the night and get through busy and hectic workdays without bingeing on sugar and caffeine. Her weight was down to 152lb, but more importantly for her she felt she had the tools to keep her weight off and maintain her progress in the long term.

Tracy's follow-up lab results 12 weeks later are shown in Figure 9.5.

Lab Test	Normal Range	Tracy's Levels	Significance
CRP-hs	Optimal less than 1.0	1.0	Cut inflammatory levels in half
Fasting Insulin	Optimal less than 50	48	Improved insulin sensitivity 2-fold
HA1c	Optimal less than 0.55	0.54	Moved into optimal range
Fructoseamine	Optimal less than 180	180	Significant reduction
Triglycerides	Optimal less than 1.00	0.98	Optimal
GGT	Less than 30	14	Optimal
Secretory IgA (stool)	50-200	146	Normal
Bacterial Culture (stool)	*Expected Flora* Bifidobacterium spp. +3-4 Lactobacillus spp. +3-4	*Expected Flora* Bifidobacterium spp. +3 Lactobacillus spp. +3	Normal
	Dysbiotic Flora None present	*Dysbiotic Flora* None	Normal

Figure 9.5. Summary of Tracy's Lab Test Results at 12 Weeks

FINAL WORD

You've now got all the tools you need to upgrade your health, lose weight and keep it off in the long term. You can expect to lose between 8-16lb of body fat over the next eight weeks, which is a fantastic result! Remember, the greater your compliance and the more accurately you adhere to the protocol, the better your results will be.

If you have a lot of weight to lose or the program outline in this chapter seems too aggressive for you, then contact us at DrBubbs.com for a modified version. Alternatively, we can help you find a qualified trainer, nutritionist or naturopath in your area.

The weight-loss process is different for each individual. You may lose weight faster or more slowly than your friends, family or colleagues. If you hit any roadblocks, revisit the principles of the Keto-Paleo dietary plan, re-assess your workout regime and retest the specific labs (see Chapter 7) to get your results headed back in the right direction.

If you've achieved your desired weight and best body, you have the luxury of several options: maintain the same eating and exercise patterns in the long term (if your new routine suits your lifestyle) or if you feel you've been restricting or limiting some enjoyable foods or treats, slowly bring them back into your diet in moderation, one day per week, as a reward for your hard work. It will take some experimentation to determine the exact amount you can re-introduce into the diet.

After you've finished the eight-week protocol, give yourself a big pat on the back! Your hard work, determination, and dedication will pay off more than you can imagine. You will have built a better brain, better body and better YOU!

CHAPTER 10

UPGRADE YOUR PERFORMANCE—
The Performance Plan

If you've completed the first eight chapters of this book, you're already well on your way to building a solid foundation for optimal performance. You've upgraded your nutrition via the Modern Paleo approach—achieving your ideal intake of protein, healthy fats, veggies and carbs.

You've also hacked your health—digestion, immunity, inflammation and hormone balance (insulin and cortisol)—and made the necessary changes to ensure your body is firing on all cylinders. Now, you've reached the peak of the *Paleo Project Pyramid* and are ready to achieve your performance potential.

I'll always remember a terrific quote I heard from a world-class strength coach Clance Laylor many years ago: *"All things being equal, the stronger athlete always wins!"* If you want to raise your game and reach a new level of strength, size and/or performance remember this mantra.

This is just as important for endurance athletes and often overlooked. If you are a cyclist, marathoner or tri-athlete this applies to you as well. The stronger you are, the more potential horsepower you have in your aerobic engine!

The term *anabolic* refers to building tissues and in this case refers to building muscle tissue. Whether you are trying to build bigger muscles, improve your 10k run time, or perform a personal best WOD (CrossFit-speak for workout of the day), shifting your body into an anabolic state is top priority. High intensity exercise or long training sessions (common in endurance sports) raise catabolic hormones, which must be tempered by an anabolic diet and supplementation plan to maximize your performance.

A mistake most people make is trying to improve their performance, while trying to get leaner. While it's possible to gain lean mass, lose body fat and improve your performance all at the same time, you'll make the most progress by focusing on only *one* goal.

Chasing two goals at opposite ends of the spectrum—performance *and* better body composition—typically leads to sub-optimal results in both. Being lean doesn't improve your deadlift; being strong doesn't necessarily give you a six-pack. In fact, getting *too lean* can hinder recovery and performance by unnecessarily raising stress hormone levels.

In this final chapter, I'll complete the *Paleo Project Pyramid*, discuss the key anabolic hormones and review my top five performance principles. I will outline a detailed diet, exercise and supplement performance plan so you can achieve your goals.

I. ANABOLIC HORMONES

Your ability to pack on muscle, lift heavier weights, and run/swim/cycle faster and farther is largely dependent on your anabolic building hormones: testosterone, insulin, and growth hormone (GH), summarized in Figure 10.1. Understanding the anabolic hormones will allow you to build muscle, strength and power more effectively and achieve your performance potential.

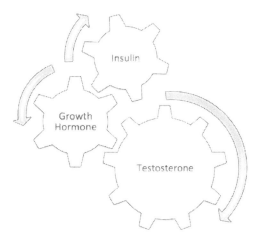

Figure 10.1. Summary of Anabolic Hormones

Testosterone

From the age of 30, your testosterone levels decrease by approximately 1% per year. Because it happens gradually most people don't realize that something is off until the symptoms become more obvious. You gain fat more easily, you're more tired in the mornings than usual, your libido is not what it once was, you don't recover as well from exercise or you don't laugh as much as you used to. These are all subtle cues that your testosterone levels are dropping.

For both men and women, testosterone is extremely important for building lean muscle mass, burning body fat, keeping your heart healthy, boosting mood and increasing libido. Studies show optimal testosterone levels in females may protect against osteoporosis. Testosterone levels will vary markedly between men and women; however, achieving the optimal level is beneficial for both sexes. Remember, optimal testosterone does *not* mean the highest possible value! You can get too much of a good thing.

Testosterone acts directly on muscle tissue to help you build lean mass and improve your overall strength. This powerful hormone is produced in the testes in men and ovaries in women and is an important marker of your anabolic potential. As a general rule, athletes engaging in intense training who have higher testosterone levels will tend to have the best results, improving both size and strength.

There are several different forms of testosterone, which are easily measured. The first measurement is *total testosterone*, accounting for 100% of your total body stores. Approximately 50% of your total testosterone is bound to a carrier protein called sex-hormone binding globulin (SHBG), which makes it unusable by the body. SHBG is important because it ensures testosterone doesn't act on all the cells it comes in contact with when travelling through your body. The remaining 50% of your total testosterone is made up of usable *bioavailable testosterone* and *free testosterone*.

Bioavailable testosterone accounts for approximately 45% of your usable testosterone; it is bound to a different carrier protein—albumin—that makes it readily absorbable. Your bioavailable testosterone levels tell you how much fuel you have in your testosterone gas tank because, unlike SHBG, albumin-bound testosterone is usable by the body.

The remaining 5% of your usable testosterone is in the unbound form called free testosterone. Free testosterone is the most biologically active form of testosterone and can be measured in conjunction with cortisol (free testosterone to cortisol ratio) to assess your total stress load or over-training.

As you age, your testosterone levels will naturally decline and SHBG levels increase, a condition more significant for men and known as *andropause*. However, you are not completely at the mercy of Father Time. By adopting the right diet, exercise and lifestyle plan, you can maximize your testosterone levels, build more muscle mass, and boost your mood and libido.

Zinc Deficiency and Testosterone

Zinc plays a major role in maintaining optimal androgen and testosterone levels in both men and women. A recent study of ten male wrestlers demonstrated that performing intense exercise to a state of exhaustion seriously depleted testosterone levels. Interestingly, athletes supplementing with zinc post-training did not experience *any reductions* in testosterone.[1]

Zinc supplementation will help to increase testosterone levels only if your levels are sub-optimal or deficient. Lab testing reveals whether or not you have a zinc deficiency. Foods naturally rich in zinc include oysters, venison, cashews and ginger root.

Sluggish Liver and Testosterone

When your liver is working hard to process such things as alcohol, fast foods, coffee, medications or recreational drugs, it gets bogged down with too much work. Your liver has many important tasks such as clearing estrogen hormones out of your body. A sluggish liver leads to the accumulation of estrogens and an unfavourable testosterone to estrogen ratio (T:E). As your T:E ratio declines, so does your anabolic potential. This can lead to symptoms of testosterone deficiency such as increased belly fat, fat accumulation around the chest for men, inability to burn fat and low libido. Lab testing for liver enzyme (ALT, GGT) levels will tell you how hard your liver is really working.

Growth Hormone

Growth hormone (GH) is your body's fountain-of-youth hormone and a powerful indicator of your anabolic potential. It helps you build lean muscle more easily and keeps your immune system robust and recovery strong. Growth hormone is made by your pituitary gland and is secreted in small bursts during deep sleep, several hours after melatonin levels have peaked. GH only remains active in the bloodstream for several minutes, making it very difficult to measure using lab tests.

In the liver, GH is converted to insulin-like growth factor-1 (IGF-1), which then exerts many of its powerful anabolic effects. Therefore, IGF-1 levels are associated with your growth hormone levels and commonly used as a reliable lab marker for GH status in the body. Optimal GH levels help you build mass, burn body fat and accelerate recovery.

Insulin

Insulin is one of your main *anabolic* switches, stimulating the body to go into building mode. When you are training intensely, a rise in insulin levels after exercise is desirable to promote the uptake of amino acids into muscle tissue and stimulate lean muscle protein synthesis.

Insulin serves another important role—it is powerfully *anti-catabolic*! This is crucial to stop the breakdown of lean muscle that happens during and after exercise. High cortisol levels trigger catabolism and muscle breakdown mode to fuel your body. If your cortisol levels stay elevated after training, you'll be breaking down precious muscle while sitting at your desk or commuting home. This will dramatically halt your progress and performance. If you're an endurance athlete pay special attention here because long training sessions (greater than 60 minutes) greatly increase your cortisol and adrenaline levels, making insulin output post-training a top priority.

When combined with optimal testosterone output from resistance training, optimal insulin sensitivity provides the ideal terrain for getting bigger and stronger. Insulin levels can be measured by lab tests, typically first thing upon rising in a fasted state.

II. PERFORMANCE PRINCIPLES

1) You Must Lift Weights

Whether you are training to improve your strength, doing a cycling time trial, running a marathon or performing on the playing field, weight training is an absolute must for men and women! Lifting weights stimulates increases in testosterone levels, crucial for getting bigger, faster or stronger.[2] In particular, endurance athletes reap the most rewards for a well-designed weight training protocol because they dismiss the gym as a tool solely for team-sport athletes or bodybuilders. Nothing could be further from the truth.

Better testosterone output translates to better mood, cardiovascular health, bone density and libido. However, if you are an elite or competitive athlete, you must guard against *over-training* because this will deplete testosterone stores and compromise performance and health.

2) You Must Perform Compound/Olympic Lifts

You need to incorporate compound exercises in order to maximize testosterone and growth hormone production during training. The major movements such as deadlifts, squats and Olympic lifts (snatch and cleans) should be performed first in your routine (after your warm up) because they produce the greatest testosterone output.[3,4] A better squat, deadlift or clean and jerk translates extremely well to better performance on the playing field or in your endurance race. CrossFit is another excellent way of packaging these types of fundamental exercises together in a way that is intense and effective. Wherever you perform these compound lifts in the gym or "in the box," you will see results.

It's important to note that strength increases are greatest when lower-body and upper-body exercises are combined in one session; therefore, be sure to start all your workouts with one or two of these compound lifts.[5] As a general rule, to maximize performance you should use barbell-based movements for *at least* the first two exercises in every training session.

3) You Must Alter Volume and Intensity

The intensity and volume of your training plays a major role in testosterone response. If you keep the intensity constant (i.e., weight on the bar), studies show that the higher volume training will elicit the greatest testosterone response. For example, a protocol of 10 sets of 10 squat repetitions at 70% of your one-repetition maximum (1RM) elicits a much greater testosterone response than 20 sets of one repetition.[6]

On the other hand, if you keep the repetitions constant, then the protocol with the greatest intensity—or weight on the bar—provides the greatest testosterone response.[7] For example, two identical protocols of three to six sets of squats will elicit the greatest testosterone response in the group lifting at 100% of 1RM compared to the group lifting at 70% of 1RM.

The best method of increasing testosterone is a moderate-intensity, high-volume approach discussed above (i.e., 10 sets of 10 reps), interspersed with heavier intensification phases (building up to your maximum lifts or 1RM) to maximize strength gains.

If you are an older athlete, have past injuries or are new to weight training (e.g., many endurance-based athletes) then starting with the lighter load is a good idea. In fact, new studies show just 50% of 1RM will raise testosterone levels dramatically at sets of 15-20 repetitions.[8] Remember to use good form for all lifts, no matter how heavy the load.

4) You Must Consume Optimal Protein and Calories

You can't build a bigger, stronger or faster athletic body without adequate raw materials. It is very common for clients and even athletes to "under eat" and assume they are consuming the right amount of protein and calories.

If you aren't getting the correct amount of raw material into your system, there is little chance you will maximize your strength, speed or size gains. Your optimal daily protein intake should be between 1.5-2.0g/kg bodyweight and your optimal caloric intake should be 50 calories/kg bodyweight.[9] (Remember, your calories should be from healthy Modern Paleo choices, such as quality fats, gluten-free "clean" carbs, and natural simple sugars). It is critical not only for building lean mass but maintaining your progress in the long run.

5) You Must Take Advantage of Nutrient Timing

Working muscles need sources of instant energy to fuel training and exercise. Before, during and after exercise are key times when consuming the right ratio of nutrients accelerates your progress and helps you break through plateaus.

The best choice *before or after exercise* is to have quickly absorbed proteins and carbohydrates in order to help you improve nutrient delivery to muscles, reduce muscle glycogen losses and limit cortisol output and muscle protein breakdown. In my Performance Plan I describe how you can take advantage of nutrient timing to achieve your goals.

III. THE PERFORMANCE PLAN

THE 3-PART PLAN

1. The Anabolic Diet

2. The Anabolic Exercise Plan

3. Performance Supplementation

To improve your performance in the gym, on the field or in the boardroom, you will need to incorporate, a personalized *anabolic* diet, anabolic exercise and performance supplementation in your regime. A summary is shown in Figure 10.2.

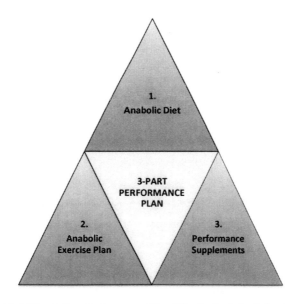

Figure 10.2. The 3-Part Performance Plan: The Peak of the Paleo Project Pyramid

My aim is to provide you with the framework from which to build better performance, regardless of whether you are a football player, avid runner, Crossfitter or simply trying to increase muscle or productivity at work. By upgrading your diet, improving your exercise regime and incorporating the right mix of supplements you can achieve your performance potential!

1) THE ANABOLIC DIET

STEP 1. ASSESS YOUR ENERGY NEEDS

You need to consume sufficient calories to account for the energy demands of your training as well as to promote lean muscle, maintain immunity and support optimal hormonal balance post-training.

In order to determine your optimal macronutrient profile—ratio of protein, fats, and carbs—you need to assess your resting metabolic rate (RMR) and degree of activity. Your RMR is the amount of energy required for you to maintain normal physiological function at rest (e.g., to keep your heart beating, lungs pumping, digestive system running, etc.). Your RMR may account for a whopping 60-70% of your daily caloric expenditure.[10]

To calculate your RMR, use the following equation:

MALES

RMR = [10 × weight (kg)] + [6.25 × height (cm)] − [5 × age (years)] + 5

EXAMPLE 1

Male, 34 years old, looking to improve physique, weighs 165lb (75kg) and stands 5'10" tall (178cm)

RMR   = (10 × 75kg) + (6.25 × 178) − (5 × 34) + 5

         = 750 + 1,112.5 − 170 +5

         = 1,688 calories per day

FEMALES

RMR = [10 × weight (kg)] + [6.25 × height (cm)] − [5 × age (years)] − 161

EXAMPLE 2

Female triathlete, 42 years old, 140lb (63.6kg) and standing 5'5" tall (165cm).

RMR   = (10 × 63.6kg) + (6.25 × 165) − (5 × 42) − 161

         = 636 + 1031 − 210 − 161

         = 1,296 calories per day

Next, you need to take into account your activity level. Simply multiply your RMR by the *Physical Activity Level (PAL)* factor listed below:

- Sedentary people (working at desk all day): multiply RMR x 1.53

- Light activity (walking or "on your feet" much of the day): multiply RMR x 1.53

- Regularly active (intense exercise three to five times a week): multiply RMR x 1.76

- Vigorously active (e.g., marathoners, triathletes, crossfitters and competitive or elite athletes): multiply RMR x 2.25

EXAMPLE 1

Regularly active male, 34 years old, weight 75kg, 178cm tall, RMR = 1,688 calories

RMR x 1.76 = Total Energy Needs

1,688 x 1.76 = Total Energy Needs

2,971 calories = Total Energy Needs Per Day

EXAMPLE 2

Vigorously active female, 42 years old, weight 63.6kg, 165cm tall, RMR = 1,296 calories

RMR x 2.25 = Total Energy Needs

1,296 x 2.25 = Total Energy Needs

2,916 calories = Total Energy Needs Per Day

STEP 2. ACHIEVE YOUR OPTIMAL PROTEIN INTAKE

Your anabolic potential is largely defined by your genetics but can be enhanced by your diet. Your first order of business when trying to add lean muscle mass or improve performance is to achieve your optimal intake of protein. If you want to get bigger, faster or stronger then it's critically important for you to consume closer to the *top end* of the 1.5-2.0g/kg bodyweight protein range. That means two grams of protein for every kilogram bodyweight. If you are trying to add lean mass, this would be for your *desired* weight, not your current weight.

For example, a 165lb (75kg) male would need to consume 113-150g of protein daily to maintain his current weight and physique. If he wants to add 15lb of muscle (total weight 180lb or 81.8kg) he needs to increase his intake to meet his *desired weight* and should be aiming for 123-164g of protein daily.

While easy to calculate, it's not always easy to put into practice. Most people overestimate their protein intake. Try calculating your total intake over a few days and you'll realize how much extra protein you need to eat to achieve your optimal intake.

Take a look at what sources of protein you *should* prioritize.

Animal Protein

You must eat *real food* protein sources if you are serious about trying to improve your performance. You'll never sustain your goals in the long term with tubs of powder. You need to get your hands dirty and learn how to cook and prepare real food!

You should prioritize supplemental protein (+ carb) shakes only around training sessions or when food preparation is not possible. There are no shortcuts to size, speed and strength; learn to eat well and the likelihood of achieving your goals will skyrocket!

Eating meat is a terrific source of essential amino acids and protein, but what most people don't realize is that meat is also the most *nutrient-dense* food—superior to vegetables, fruit, grains, beans and legumes.

Not only does it provide you with the most bioavailable protein sources, it's also a rich source of essential vitamins, minerals and important nutrients.

Milk—The Best Anabolic Liquid Food

Milk is the original post-workout protein shake, traditionally considered one of the best natural food sources for building muscle mass. Although milk contains sub-optimal amounts of muscle building BCAAs and a slower absorption rate, it still comes out on top in terms of anabolic power (neck and neck with whey isolate). Experts believe milk's ability to increase lean mass and improve recovery has to do with its ability to boost insulin release (despite a low glycemic index), its complex array of proteins and growth factors, and the presence of carbohydrates.[9]

Milk is a controversial topic in the Paleo world. If you have a lactose or casein allergy (remember, you might not know until you remove it from your diet), you'll need to eliminate milk from your sports nutrition arsenal. If you are lean and can tolerate milk, definitely include it as your post-training drink of choice.

In general, if your body-fat level is greater than approximately 12% for males and 20% in females, it's best to forego the milk and use whey protein isolate after exercise to avoid excessive gains in body fat that could compromise performance.

Whey Isolate—The Best Anabolic Supplement

Whey protein isolate is the king of protein supplements, outperforming all other protein mixtures when it comes to promoting lean muscle, strength, power and recovery.[11, 12] It even outperforms milk in some studies! Remember, although grass-fed whey *concentrate* (not whey isolate) is very healthy for you, it does *not* perform as well as whey isolate around bouts of exercise. Be sure to include whey isolate before, during and/or after training!

Remember, once you've achieved your optimal protein intake, more is not better! Your total caloric intake from fats and carbs is the next most crucial factor in optimizing your performance and achieving your goals.

STEP 3. ACHIEVE YOUR OPTIMAL FAT INTAKE

In Chapter 2, I described how fats should make up approximately 30% of your total caloric intake. This should be evenly distributed between saturated (10%), monounsaturated (10%), and polyunsaturated fats (10%).

For example, a 42-year-old female triathlete on an approximately 2,900-calorie diet would need to consume 30% (870 calories) from fats. This amounts to a total daily intake of 97g (2,900 calories x 30% = 870 calories, divided by 9kcal/gram for fats = 96.6g) or approximately two tablespoons (30g) of saturated, monounsaturated *and* polyunsaturated fats per day.

A rough estimate is for men to include at least two "thumb" sizes of fats at each meal, while women should aim for at least one "thumb." Refer to Chapter 2 for a full list of all healthy fats.

Remember, saturated fats are not just calories; they also play a crucial role in maintaining sex hormone production. Pre-exercise concentrations of testosterone are highly correlated with your total intake of fats, in particular healthy saturated and monounsaturated fats.[13] If you're following a low-fat or low-calorie diet, you will be at much greater risk of suffering from low testosterone levels. Not a great recipe for high performance!

STEP 4. ACHIEVE YOUR OPTIMAL CARB INTAKE

Now that you have calculated your total protein and fat intake, round out the rest of your caloric intake with carbohydrates. Our triathlete from the previous example is already consuming 96g of fat per day (870 calories) and, supposing she is eating her optimal daily protein intake of 128g (512 calories), she needs to consume approximately

1,534 calories (384g) of carbs during the day to achieve her 2,916 calorie diet.

This is equally important if you are trying to add lean mass and improve your physique. Most clients focus solely on increasing protein intake and don't realize you ALSO need to achieve 50 calories/kg bodyweight to support increased muscle growth and hypertrophy.[9] The right mix of fats and carbs will help you make up the difference.

As described in Chapter 3, *two-thirds* of your carb intake should be from complex carbohydrates and *one-third* from natural simple sugars. For our triathlete, this would amount to 249g of complex carbs (two-thirds of her 374g total carb intake) and 125g of simple sugars daily (one-third of her 374g total carb intake), preferably spread equally *before (42g), during (42g)* and *after (42g)* exercise to maximize adaptations to training. (This carb distribution can be modified depending on the athlete's digestive tolerance to shakes and liquid nutrition before and during exercise.)

STEP 5. NUTRIENT TIMING

Let's take a closer look at how you can prioritize your food intake around training to accelerate your progress.

Nutrient Timing—Before Exercise

Did you know that your *pre-exercise* nutrition is just as important (perhaps even *more* important) as your post-training nutrition? Recent studies show significant improvements in muscle protein synthesis with *pre-workout* supplementation of carbohydrate + protein shake compared to consuming them only post-training.[14, 15] Whey protein isolate is the best choice to take an hour before training. If you are using a vegan/vegetarian protein, ensure it has a minimum of 3g of leucine per shake (if necessary, add BCAAs to make up the difference.)

What if you are pressed for time and can't drink a shake before training? Try using an essential amino acid formula. Studies show a pre-exercise *essential amino acid (EAA)* + *dextrose* formula performed better when taken before versus after your workout.[16] It's easy, time efficient (simply add a scoop to water) and it works!

If performance is your goal, then including carbs in your pre-workout drink is absolutely essential. The desired ratio of carbs to protein is 1:1 to 4:1, depending on the individual and your sport. Low pre-exercise glycogen stores have been consistently shown to reduce performance in athletes.[17] Nothing kills an intense workout faster than an inadequate fuel supply.

Nutrient Timing—During Exercise

No matter whether you are training for team sports or endurance events, the *peri-workout* or *during* workout nutrient timing window is critical to improving performance. If you are taking a protein shake before exercise, you may be wondering why you should bother consuming another shake during your training? Researchers recently discovered that *even in a fed* state, the combination of carbohydrate + protein during training stimulated lean muscle protein during exercise.[18] In short, a carb + protein shake (1:1 to 4:1) is crucial for getting bigger, stronger or faster!

Peri-workout nutrition helps to slow glycogen loss, limit delayed onset muscle soreness (DOMS), and blunt cortisol output. These are powerful performance advantages:

i) Limit Glycogen Loss

As the intensity of exercise increases, so does your reliance on carbohydrates and muscle glycogen stores for fuel. Strength training in the gym depletes muscle glycogen levels particularly in the 8-12 repetition range compared to lower rep workouts.[19] These numbers are significantly higher during compound movements. By consuming high-glycemic carbohydrates during training you can limit the degree of glycogen depletion experienced during exercise.

For endurance athletes this is even more crucial, as your performance is directly related to glycogen stores. Fail to supply adequate carbohydrates during exercise and your glycogen losses will accelerate and your performance will plummet. Endurance athletes will always tend toward suboptimal glycogen status due to the longer nature of their training bouts.

ii) Limit DOMS

Refuelling with a protein + carbohydrate drink during exercise helps to reduce delayed onset muscle soreness (DOMS) after training. A study in the journal *Strength and Conditioning* of 34 men performing seven exercises—three sets of eight repetitions each—found considerable reductions in blood levels of myoglobin and creatine kinase (markers for muscle damage) in athletes drinking a protein + carbohydrate mixture.[20]

The journal *Medicine & Science in Sports & Exercise* showed that the consumption of a protein + carbohydrate drink during training helps you to recover for up to 24 hours post-training.[21] This is crucial for team-sport athletes, endurance athletes, Crossfitters and anyone trying to increase muscle mass because reduced muscle damage permits greater training volume and thus greater training gains.

iii) Limit Cortisol Output

Cortisol levels naturally increase during training in order to breakdown muscle tissue to fuel exercise. Excessive output during or after exercise leads to continued muscle breakdown well after you are finished training. Consuming a *peri-workout* protein + carb shake greatly reduces high cortisol levels after training, so you can preserve your precious muscle and improve recovery.[20]

Your best bet is to consume quickly absorbed proteins (such as pharmaceutical grade amino acids, whey protein isolates or hydrosylates) and add high-glycemic glucose sources such as maltodextrin, dextrose or brown rice syrup. This combination promotes a more anabolic state, mitigates cortisol output, increases lean muscle and helps maintain overall immunity.[22]

Remember, avoid consuming large amounts of fructose during exercise because it slows the rate at which food leaves your stomach (gastric emptying rate), leading to cramps, bloating and abdominal discomfort. If drinking shakes during exercise bloats you, try using an essential amino acid or BCAA formula mixed with simple carbs during your workouts.

Nutrient Timing—After Training

The goal in post-training is to mitigate the catabolic effects of exercise—elevated cortisol levels, accelerated muscle and glycogen breakdown, lowered immunity and decreased testosterone output—and promote an anabolic environment as quickly as possible.

If you are hitting the gym or CrossFit four or more times per week, training for an endurance event (marathon, triathlon, cycling race), performing two-a-day training sessions, or competing in sports 12 months of the year (with no real off-season), you'll be treading a fine line between optimal training and over-training.

If you fail to consume the necessary macronutrients—proteins, carbs and fats—after exercise you may experience the following:

- Prolonged muscle soreness

- Fatigue

- Low mood

- Increased susceptibility to colds and flu

- Low testosterone levels

- High cortisol levels

- Decreased lean mass

- Slower metabolic rate

- Poor performance in training and competition

The ingestion of high-glycemic carbohydrates and fast-absorbed proteins (1:1 to 4:1) after exercise helps to attenuate this catabolic process by stimulating the release of insulin. Insulin is a powerful anti-catabolic hormone that inhibits the breakdown of protein and lowers elevated cortisol levels.[23]

There are a couple of options for post-training nutrition:

i) Milk—Post-training

If your digestive system can handle it, milk is a great post-workout option. The journal *Medicine & Science in Sports & Exercise* compared the effects of post-exercise full-fat milk, skim milk or a placebo drink on lean mass gains. The full-fat milk group showed the greatest use of amino acids compared to the skim milk and placebo groups, resulting in greater lean muscle mass gains.[24] (Amazingly, they got leaner as well!)

Remember, milk is *not* a good choice *pre-train*ing due to its insulin-spiking effects or if you are trying to shed body fat and get leaner.

ii) Whey Isolate—Post-training

The research is very clear that whey protein isolate—compared to whey concentrate, casein, soy and rice protein—should be your top choice post-workout. Whey protein isolate supplementation increases your physical performance, muscle mass, hypertrophy, strength and recovery.[9, 25] These effects are due to its high bioavailability, high concentration of leucine (BCAA) and fast absorption rate. Pretty impressive!

ARE YOU A HARD GAINER?

Do you struggle to add muscle mass or want to upgrade your performance? Try adding *protein pulsing* to your repertoire. How does it work? After exercise, muscle protein synthesis remains elevated for approximately three hours. After this time your muscle building machinery tapers off, despite blood amino acids levels remaining elevated above normal levels.

By consuming multiple post-workout shakes after training (the first shake *immediately after* exercise, the second shake *three to four hours later*) you can ramp up muscle building a second time after the initial window comes to a close. This provides you with the additional protein and calories needed to achieve your desired lean mass or endurance performance gains.[26]

PRE-EXERCISE

•**OPTION 1: 1 HOUR BEFORE EXERCISE**
- Protein: 30-40g men; 20-30g women. Whey isolate, whey hydrosylates and/or vegan protein *(no milk)*.
- Carbs: honey, maple syrup, molasses, maltodextrin, dextrose brown rice syrup and/or fruit.

•**OPTION 2: 30 MIN OR LESS BEFORE EXERCISE**
- Essential amino acid formula (6g) + simple sugars (10-40g).

DURING EXERCISE

•**OPTION 1: WHEY OR VEGAN PROTEIN**
- Protein: 30-40g men; 20-30g women. Whey isolate, whey hydrosylates and/or vegan protein *(no milk)*.
- Carbs: honey, maple syrup, molasses, maltodextrin, dextrose brown rice syrup and/or fruit.

•**OPTION 2: AMINO ACIDS**
- Protein: EAA (6g) or BCAA (3-5g Leucine).
- Carbs: honey, maple syrup, molasses, maltodextrin, dextrose brown rice syrup and/or fruit.

AFTER EXERCISE

•**OPTION 1: A SINGLE SHAKE**
- Protein: 30-40g men; 20-30g women. Milk, whey isolate, whey hydrosylates and/or vegan protein.
- Carbs: honey, maple syrup, molasses, maltodextrin, dextrose brown rice syrup and/or fruit.

•**OPTION 2: PROTEIN PULSING** *(two post-workout shakes)*
for greater lean mass gains or "hard gainers".
- 1st shake immediately after exercise (same as Option #1)
- 2nd shake 3-4 hours after training.

Figure 10.3. Nutrient Timing For Performance—Summary Chart

2) THE ANABOLIC EXERCISE PLAN

Now that you've supercharged your nutrition to maximize your anabolic potential, it's time to do the same with your training. Let's start with the more elite or high-performing athletes. Entire books have been written on training programs for adding lean muscle, strength and power in sports such as football, baseball, CrossFit, endurance sports, etc. It would be impossible to write a single program to meet the needs of all these populations.

With this in mind, if you are *already* training at a high level (with appropriate coaching) and you are still not achieving your performance potential, you likely have deficiencies in your performance nutrition (go back to Step 1. The Anabolic Diet) or supplementation protocol (see below, 3. Performance Supplementation). A key system in your body may also be imbalanced or dysfunctional (go back to Section II and ensure you *passed* all self-assessments).

If you are not working with a highly qualified trainer and want to increase your strength and lean muscle mass for better performance or improved health, I have included an anabolic exercise routine in *Appendix D* for you to start your journey.

The best way to overcome plateaus in your training or performance is to simplify things and bring your focus back to your primary goal. The more clearly you define it, the clearer your roadmap and the quicker your success.

In my experience, combining weight training with sprint training is the fastest way to get yourself fit, strong and ready to perform your best, regardless of whether you are an endurance athlete, hockey player or trying to qualify for CrossFit Games.

STRENGTH TRAINING

Did you know that renowned Olympic lifting coach Pierre Roy uses only about 12 different exercises with his world-class Olympic athletes? If you take into account that many of his exercises are variations of the same movements (cleans, snatches and squats), he really only uses a handful of exercises to build the strongest and most athletic bodies in the world! If that's all they need, surely the rest of us can benefit from a simpler approach.

I like to use a modified version of *German Volume Training*, a high-volume approach to exercise that triggers greater testosterone output, lean muscle mass and strength. Studies show that performing 10 sets of 10 repetitions at 70% of your 1RM (maximum) leads to significant elevations in testosterone.[6] If you are a novice trainee or new to weight lifting, you may only need to use 50% of your 1RM to induce increases in testosterone.[8]

See *Appendix D* for full details on the key strength exercises you should perform. Always start your training sessions by performing lower body exercises first, as they produce the greatest testosterone response. Also, be sure to include both lower body and upper body exercises every session because this translates to greater strength increases.

It's important to remember that regardless of your sport (tennis, hockey, basketball, etc.), or your endurance event (marathon, triathlon, cycling) lifting weights will accelerate your progress in a big way! Remember, the strongest athlete always wins and my goal here is to make you stronger and more athletic.

HIIT TRAINING

Sprinting is tremendously advantageous for just about every sport. Whether you are a baseball player, marathoner, hockey player, Crossfitter or triathlete you will improve your performance by adding sprinting to your repertoire. The benefits of HIIT and sprinting include:

- Improved athleticism

- Improved anaerobic conditioning

- Increased fast-twitch fibre activity

- Increased force production

- Increased endurance and work capacity

- Improved cardiovascular health

- Improved insulin sensitivity

- Improved cognition and brain volume

It would be difficult to select another exercise that increases all these important factors to the same degree. As these parameters improve, so will your performance on the bike, in the gym, "in the box" or on the playing field. Of course, they should be applied in conjunction with your sport-specific training regime. Ideally, perform the sprints outside on a track or grass. (Your next best option indoors is on a stationary bike.) See Appendix E for the full program.

You can try adding some *Energy Systems* training sessions using farmer's walks, sled drags and prowler pushes to simulate HIIT and improve your conditioning. Not sure what those things are? Check out Dr.Bubbs.com to find out what you are missing!

CASE STUDY #1—CROSSFIT PERFORMANCE

Rajvir, a 27-year-old salesman and Crossfitter came to me with complaints of intense fatigue, inability to shed body fat, and poor performance during recent CrossFit WODs. He regularly consumed multiple cups of coffee at work and before training, but felt he lacked the spark that he normally experienced during training. He couldn't push himself through difficult sessions and his work output had significantly declined. Rajvir also had difficulty staying asleep over the past three months, something he had not experienced in the past.

Rajvir was exhibiting some classic signs of overtraining: excessive stress response, poor recovery, depressed mood and irritability, and strong cravings for sweets and salt. His lab tests revealed what you see in Figure 10.4.

Lab Test	Normal Range	Rajvir's Levels	Significance
WBC	4-11	3.5	Low – possibly due to stress or infection
Free Testosterone (Blood)	30-95	24	Low – acutely rundown or fatigued
Cortisol (Blood)	150-720	330	Low – possible under-performing adrenals
Free T/Cortisol Ratio	0.12-0.20	0.07	Low – acutely rundown or fatigued
DHEA	2-10	3.0	Low Normal – moderately long-term stress response
HA1c	0.040-0.060	0.057	High Normal – sub-optimal blood sugar control
Urinalysis - Specific Gravity (SG)	Ideal 1.005-1.015	1.030	High – dehydrated

Figure 10.4. Summary of Rajvir's Lab Test Results

His low white blood cell (WBC) count and low free testosterone levels supported my suspicion that Rajvir had been overtraining. Rajvir had assumed he needed more training to offset his poor performance; however, his lab results revealed he needed to be more efficient with his training and he needed more rest! A urinalysis showed he was significantly dehydrated, due to his excessive coffee consumption and heavy reliance on pre-workout caffeine pills over the past three months.

In the next four weeks he eliminated all stimulants. Rajvir was heavily taxing his sympathetic nervous system, and the excessive caffeine intake was disrupting his sleep and compromising recovery. In addition, his diet was not good enough for a high performing crossfitter. He increased his protein intake to 2g per kilogram bodyweight and boosted his saturated fat intake substantially. Rajvir was worried this would lead to increased body fat, but I explained to him that his high intake of processed sugars (candy) during late night binges was more detrimental to his health and performance. He also mildly reduced his carbohydrate intake and shifted the majority before and after his training bouts to maximize glycogen uptake and support healthy fat loss throughout the day. Finally, I added some herbal supplementation to correct his adrenal dysfunction.

After ten days, Rajvir's intense sugar cravings had subsided and his evening candy binges were now gone. He felt satiated throughout the day on the keto-Paleo diet due to the higher protein and fat intake. After four weeks, he had no trouble falling asleep, had dropped 4% body fat, and felt strong again during his CrossFit training sessions. Rajvir was very pleased four weeks later, when he performed multiple personal best WODs!

3) PERFORMANCE SUPPLEMENTATION

Today, training in the gym or during the off-season is not the same as in the past. The intensity and complexity of the workout regimes is much greater, producing stronger, fitter and faster athletes. Gone are the days of binging during the off-season and relying on your talent and genetics alone to get the job done.

Athletes place more demands on their bodies than in previous generations. It's no accident that many of today's top athletes are performing at a high level well into their 30s and 40s, something unheard of in generations past. Better nutrition plans, exercise protocols and performance supplementation supports accelerated recovery and rebuilding of the body.

In order to take your training and performance to the next level, you may need to add some targeted supplementation to get the job done. While the store shelves are lined with endless supplements with exaggerated claims for improving performance, there are really only a handful you need to upgrade your performance and support superior recovery.

There are three supplements in particular that have proven results when it comes to enhancing performance: creatine, caffeine and leucine (BCAA or Whey).

CREATINE

Creatine is a naturally occurring amino acid (composed of three smaller amino acids —arginine, glycine and methionine) that is produced in your muscle tissue, liver and pancreas. You can obtain it from your diet because it's abundantly found in red meat and fish.

Creatine is the *most* highly researched sports supplement on the marketplace. How does it work? It is converted to creatine phosphate in muscle tissue, where it's used as a high-energy compound during weight lifting or quick explosive movements. Your alactic anaerobic energy system (movements less than 10 seconds) uses the high-energy creatine phosphate to produce ATP (adenosine triphosphate), the primary energy currency of your body. The more ATP you can produce quickly, the more power you have. This translates into greater adaptations to training and superior performance on the playing field.

Your naturally occurring creatine stores are typically 60-70% of what your body is capable of storing. Supplementing with creatine completely saturates your muscles stores (100%), allowing you to produce more ATP and maximize your power and strength potential.

Creatine supplementation has been shown to increase maximal strength, strength endurance, muscle hypertrophy and lean mass in conjunction with sprinting, heavy resistance training or plyometrics.[27] No matter what your sport, this will translate into better results (even for endurance athletes, more on this below.) Anecdotal side effects of creatine supplementation have included muscle cramps, dehydration, increased incidence of injury and possible liver or kidney damage. These claims are *not* supported by the latest research, providing dosing is correct.[28]

If you want to add creatine to your supplement regime, add 5g daily over 10-12 weeks.[29, 30] Creatine is best absorbed when insulin levels are elevated, so post-training supplementation along with a carbohydrate plus protein drink, or at mealtime, is highly recommended.[31]

Creatine and Endurance Exercise

Creatine supplementation in endurance athletes has often been regarded as an afterthought due to the aerobic nature of the sport. However, new research shows creatine considerably improves repetitive high intensity sprint intervals, providing endurance athletes with important and highly advantageous training adaptations. In addition, creatine improves work capacity and recovery, additional benefits that endurance athletes can use to maximize performance.[25]

CAFFEINE

Caffeine is a natural central nervous system stimulant that exerts numerous potential benefits in terms of performance. It helps you improve work capacity and body composition by mobilizing your body-fat stores to be burned for energy. More importantly, it does so while sparing your precious muscle glycogen stores, a tremendous potential athletic advantage.[32]

If you can use fat for fuel while preserving glycogen, you'll be able to increase your work capacity and sustain higher performance over a longer period of time. This is an incredible advantage for endurance sports, CrossFit, and intense strength training sessions. (Recall that glycogen depletion is directly related to reduced work capacity during high-intensity exercise.)

Caffeine typically takes 15-30 minutes to be metabolized by the liver and make its way into your bloodstream, reaching peak concentrations after one hour.[33] Supplementing with caffeine actually yields *greater improvements* in endurance and time to exhaustion compared to getting your caffeine hit from drinking coffee.[34,35]

If performance is your top priority, add a caffeine supplement. Take 150-200mg of caffeine 30-60 minutes before training to boost your training results. If you want to get more specific with your intake, you can increase to 3-9mg/kg of bodyweight prior to exercise. Do not exceed this level—allowable levels set by the International Olympic Committee are approximately 12 mcg/mL.[25, 32]

Alternatively, if you're a coffee lover and don't mind the mild performance deficit then you can stick with your pre-workout coffee. However, be mindful not to over consume caffeine because it can lead to fatigue, poor recovery, feeling run down, disturbed sleep, depressed immunity and lower testosterone levels. Studies show habitual coffee drinkers do not get the same level of benefit as non-regular coffee drinkers when it comes to training response.[36] Moderation is the key to maximizing the benefits and mitigating the risks of caffeine.

Another option is to incorporate *caffeine cycling,* which is altering your caffeine intake from week to week, just as you do with training. The following is a sample month:

Caffeine Cycling

Week 1 – Espresso (80mg of caffeine per day)

Week 2 – Regular cup of coffee (12oz, 120-150mg caffeine per day)

Week 3 – Two cups of coffee (240-300mg caffeine per day)

Week 4 – TAPER – No coffee, or one cup of green tea (30-40mg caffeine)

By cycling your caffeine intake, you can maximize the benefits of caffeine without de-sensitizing yourself and limiting the benefits. Remember, drink all caffeinated beverages before noon to avoid disrupting deep sleep and recovery.

BETA-ALANINE AND PERFORMANCE

If your favourite sport relies primarily on the lactic energy system, you could gain a significant edge from supplementing with the amino acid beta-alanine. How can this help your 10k run, CrossFit training or next soccer game? Let me review.

Carnosine is a dipeptide protein found primarily in fast-twitch muscle fibres. It supports better performance by buffering the accumulation of hydrogen ions (H+) in your muscle tissue, helping you to clear the burn you feel when exercising or lifting weights.

You may be wondering where beta-alanine fits into this picture. The production of carnosine depends on the amount of beta-alanine present in your muscle cells. By supplementing with beta-alanine, you can increase carnosine levels in your muscles and buffer the build-up of lactic acid during training. This translates to better performance on the playing field and in the gym.

Supplementing with beta-alanine during HIIT training is a terrific combination. Researchers at the University of Oklahoma investigated the effects of beta-alanine supplementation on HIIT training over six weeks. Those cyclists supplementing with beta-alanine improved their endurance performance and increased lean muscle mass.[37,38,39] Better performance and a better body—impressive results! The optimal dose of beta-alanine ranges between 3-6g daily, depending on the athlete. Note: Symptoms of paresthesia—a sensation of tingling, burning or numbness of your skin—may be experienced at doses greater than 1g, so start low and go slow. Alternatively, time-release formulas or multiple doses throughout the day should be considered.

LEUCINE (WHEY, EAA, OR BCAA)

Leucine is the all-star amino acid of the branched-chain amino acids for its ability to up-regulate important genetic pathways that control muscle building. Studies show that leucine supplementation provides serious performance benefits: [40, 41, 42]

- Increased muscle protein synthesis

- Improved exercise capacity

- Increased muscular power and endurance

- Reduced post-exercise soreness

- Improved immune function

A standard serving of protein typically contains only 5-10% leucine, making supplementation with BCAA, EAA or whey a key component of any performance supplementation protocol. Studies consistently show considerable decreases in blood levels of leucine following aerobic (15 to 33%), anaerobic lactic (10%) and strength-training (30%) sessions.[25]

In Japan, a recent study examined the effects of BCAA supplementation on the lactate threshold, a well-accepted measure of exercise capacity. The athletes who consumed a BCAA drink with higher leucine content demonstrated increased exercise capacity and endurance at lactate threshold.[43] Improved exercise capacity translates into better performance during training or competition especially for team-sports athletes, endurance competitors and Crossfitters!

In Australia, a study examined the effects of leucine supplementation on muscular power production in canoeists. Competitive outrigger canoeists were divided into two groups, half taking a leucine supplement and the other half a placebo. Research results showed that those subjects consuming the leucine supplement dramatically increased muscular power production after six weeks of supplementation compared to the placebo.[42] Top strength coaches all agree that greater power production translates into greater success on the playing field!

BCAAs not only help improve exercise endurance and muscular power, they actually help minimize muscular damage after prolonged exercise. A study at *Sacred Heart University in Connecticut* showed that lactate dehydrogenase (LDH) levels—a marker for muscular damage—was considerably reduced in athletes supplementing with BCAAs.[44] Again, athletes performing two-a-day training sessions, CrossFit trainees and endurance athletes would benefit greatly from this effect.

Finally, in Chapter 5 I discussed how athletes training intensely often have depleted immunity. In Italy, sports scientists found that BCAA supplementation not only reduces muscle soreness, but also *improves immune function*.[45] Study participants showed increased plasma glutamine levels, recovered mononuclear cell proliferation and modified exercise-related cytokine response, all of which are important markers for improved immune function.

CASE STUDY #2—INCREASING LEAN MUSCLE MASS

Tyler, a 28-year-old computer programmer, had recently taken up weight lifting and was determined to bulk up and add muscle mass. He weighed 155lb and was looking to add 10 pounds of muscle to his frame. He had hit a plateau one year into his training and was wondering how to get things back on track to achieve his goals.

After reviewing Tyler's dietary regime, there were a couple of shortcomings. First, it was evident he was not taking in enough protein. While he had done a great job of improving his diet over the past year, he had underestimated just how much protein he needed to add that extra muscle. He bumped up his intake to 160g, divided into three meals + one shake over the course of the day.

Next, he wasn't taking in enough calories. To correct this, Tyler dramatically increased his carbohydrate intake after training as well as his fat intake through the day. Lastly, he added a coffee before his morning workouts (previously he drank only tea), BCAA supplementation during training, and added 5g of creatine supplementation daily.

On the exercise front, he switched his twice-weekly aerobic runs to two bouts of sprints (HIIT) to develop more posterior chain (glutes, hamstrings) strength, which carried over well to the gym. Check out Tyler's results in Figure 10.4 after eight weeks on the protocol.

	Weight	Lean Muscle	Fat Mass	% Fat	Bioavailable Testosterone
Starting	155 lbs.	136	19 lbs.	12%	4.5
After 8 Weeks	164 lbs.	148	16 lbs.	10%	8.5
Change	↑ 9 lbs.	↑ 12 lbs.	↓ 3 lbs.	↓ 2%	↑ Almost DOUBLE!

Figure 10.5. Summary of Tyler's Results After Eight Weeks

Tyler knocked it out of the park! He changed his diet (admitting afterwards he almost couldn't get through that much food!), upgraded his training routine and reaped the rewards of his hard work. The best part is that one year later, during our annual follow-up visit, he was at 165 pounds and still 10% body fat. He had found the sweet spot with his diet and exercise routine and confessed he actually found it easy to maintain now!

FINAL WORD

Congratulations, you made it to the peak of the Paleo Project Pyramid!

You've upgraded your nutrition via the Modern Paleo diet to meet the rigorous demands of your training and work schedule. You've hacked your health and upgraded key systems of your body—digestion, immunity, inflammation, and hormones insulin and cortisol. And now you have the roadmap for achieving your performance potential.

Remember, for some people the changes will be immediate, while for others it may take a little longer. Prioritize the areas in Section I and II where you need more support, stick with the game plan provided, take a step-by-step approach and you will reap the benefits in the long run.

If you already train in a specific sport, simply add the appropriate layers of the *Paleo Project Pyramid*—upgrading nutrition and hacking your health—to help you correct deficiencies and imbalances, and augment your performance with your Three-Step Performance Plan: the anabolic diet, the anabolic exercise plan, and performance supplementation.

Best of luck on your journey to better health and performance! Your hard work and dedication will allow you to reach new heights in the gym, during competition and in all other aspects of your life. Once you've achieved your performance goals, track your health markers to monitor your growth and improvement from year to year.

Remember, don't set limitations on your mind or body. Believe it and you can achieve it! There is no greater feeling than overcoming mental and physical plateaus that have held you back for years. My hope is that the *Paleo Project* played a role in helping get you there. *Best of luck on your journey!*

APPENDIX A

HCL CHALLENGE PROTOCOL

Day 1
- Take one capsule of Betaine HCl + Pepsin after the first few bites of your biggest meal of the day.

- Wait to see if you notice a warm feeling in your chest or throat after the meal.

    - If you feel a warm sensation, discontinue HCl Challenge.

    - If you do not feel a warm sensation, proceed to Day 2.

Day 2
- Take two capsules of Betaine HCl + Pepsin after the first few bites of your biggest meal of the day.

- Wait to see if you notice a warm feeling in your chest or throat after the meal.

    - If you feel a warm sensation, reduce to one capsule as your daily maintenance dose. The HCl Challenge is now complete.

    - If you do not feel a warm sensation, proceed to Day 3.

Day 3

- Take three capsules of Betaine HCl + Pepsin after the first few bites of your biggest meal of the day.

- Wait to see if you notice a warm feeling in your chest or throat after the meal.

    - If you feel a warm sensation, reduce to two capsules as your daily maintenance dose. The HCl Challenge is now complete.

    - If you do not feel a warm sensation, proceed to Day 4.

Continue this process until you reach a maximum of six capsules, or you feel the warm sensation.

Notes:

- Do not exceed six capsules per day, unless advised by a health-care professional.

- It is not uncommon to get up to or very close to the maximum dose.

- Your maintenance dose is the number of capsules you will take once per day at your biggest meal. You will continue at this dose until you:

    i.   Finish the bottle of HCl + Pepsin, or

    ii. Feel the warm sensation, at which point reduce your maintenance dose by one capsule (e.g., from four to three caps)

- If you remain stuck on four capsules or higher, contact your local naturopath or functional doctor to examine other causes of poor digestion.

Warning: Betain HCL and Pepsin should not be used concurrently with H2-blocking drugs and proton pump inhibitors (PPI) because these drugs are intended to block the production of stomach acid.

APPENDIX B

BEGINNER HIIT PROTOCOL

To start, find a nearby track or simply pace off the desired distance in your local park or a quiet street. At the beginning of each session, warm-up gently for three to five minutes with a light jog. Then, you sprint!

Here is your plan for the next eight weeks. Perform each workout *twice* weekly:

Phase I

WEEK	WORKOUT (Sets x Distance)	REST PERIOD
1	5 x 50m	60s
2	6 x 50m	60s
3	8 x 50m	60s
4	10 x 50m	60s

Phase II

WEEK	WORKOUT (Sets x Distance)	REST PERIOD
5	5 x 100m	60s
6	6 x 100m	60s
7	8 x 100m	60s
8	10 x 100m	60s

APPENDIX C

STRENGTH TRAINING FOR FAT LOSS & BODY COMPOSITION

Check out DrBubbs.com to review the proper form and technique for each movement.

Day 1 Routine

A1) Goblet Squats – 2-3 sets x 15 reps (Rest – 0s)
A2) DB Rows (Elbow In) – 2-3 sets x 15 reps each side (Rest – 0s)
A3) Front Planks – 2-3 sets x max time (Rest – 30s)

B1) Split Squats – 2-3 sets x 10 reps each side (Rest – 0s)
B2) Cable Rows (Elbows Out) – 2-3 sets x 15 reps (Rest – 0s)
B3) Side Planks – 2-3 sets x max time each (Rest – 30s)

C1) Hip Thrust – 2-3 sets x 15-20 reps (Rest – 0s)
C2) DB Tricep Extension – 2-3 sets x 15 reps (Rest – 0s)
C3) DB Lateral Raise + External Rotation
– 2-3 sets x 15 reps (Rest – 30s)

Day 2 Routine

A1) DB Deadlifts – 2-3 sets x 15 reps (Rest – 0s)

A2) DB Chest Press – 2-3 sets x 15 reps (Rest – 0s)

A3) Half Kneeling Chop – 2-3 sets x 12 reps each side (Rest – 30s)

B1) Lateral Lunges – 2-3 sets x 10 reps per leg (Rest – 0s)

B2) DB Pullover – 2-3 sets x 15 reps (Rest – 0s)

B3) Lower Abs – DeadBug – 2-3 sets x 10-20 reps (Rest – 30s)

C1) Hip Thrust (1-leg) – 2-3 sets x 15-20 reps (Rest – 0s)

C2) DB Bicep Curl – 2-3 sets x 15 reps (Rest – 0s)

C3) DB External Rotation (Side Lying) – 2-3
sets x 15 reps each (Rest – 30s)

APPENDIX D

THE ANABOLIC EXERCISE PLAN

Check out DrBubbs.com for free videos demonstrating the following exercises.

Beginner Program: Strength Training
Day 1 (Monday)

A1) Deadlifts	Sets x Reps	Intensity	Rest
Week 1	5 x 10	50% 1RM	60s
Week 2	6 x 10	50% 1RM	60s
Week 3	8 x 10	50% 1RM	60s
Week 4	10 x 10	50% 1RM	60s

Note: if you are able to complete all sets for 10 repetitions, increase the weight on the bar by 10%.

If you do not know your 1RM, use a weight you are comfortable with for 15 repetitions.

B1) Bench Press	Sets x Reps	Intensity	Rest
Week 1	5 x 10	60% 1RM	60s
Week 2	6 x 10	60% 1RM	60s
Week 3	8 x 10	60% 1RM	60s
Week 4	10 x 10	60% 1RM	60s

Note: if you are able to complete all sets for 10 repetitions, increase the weight on the bar by 5%.

If you do not know your 1RM, use a weight you are comfortable with for 15 repetitions.

C1) Supplementary Exercise	Reps	Rest
Choose one exercise from LIST A	3 x 10-12	0s

C2) Supplementary Exercise	Reps	Rest
Choose one exercise from LIST B	3 x 10-12	0s

Choose one of the following exercises from each list, perform three sets of 10-12 reps. Select a different exercise for each training day.

List A

1. Cable Row – Rope (Elbow Out)

2. Face Pull – Rope

3. DB Row – Single-Arm (Elbow Out)

4. DB Pullover

List B

1. Seated External Rotation DB

2. Scarecrows DB

3. Lateral Raise + External Rotation DB

4. Band Pull Apart

Beginner Program

Day 2 (Thursday)

A1) Squats	Sets x Reps	Intensity	Rest
Week 1	5 x 10	50% 1RM	60s
Week 2	6 x 10	50% 1RM	60s
Week 3	8 x 10	50% 1RM	60s
Week 4	10 x 10	50% 1RM	60s

Note: if you are able to complete all sets for 10 repetitions, increase the weight on the bar by 10%.

If you do not know your 1RM, use a weight you are comfortable with for 15 repetitions.

B1) Lat Pulldown (Underhand Grip)	Sets x Reps	Intensity	Rest
Week 1	5 x 10	★	60s
Week 2	6 x 10	★	60s
Week 3	8 x 10	★	60s
Week 4	10 x 10	★	60s

Note: use a weight you are comfortable with for 15 repetitions. If you are able to complete all sets for 10 repetitions, increase the weight on the bar by 5%.

C1) Supplementary Exercise	Reps	Rest
Choose one exercise from LIST A	3 x 10-12	0s

C2) Supplementary Exercise	Reps	Rest
Choose one exercise from LIST B	3 x 10-12	0s

Choose from the exercises in List A and List B on page 242. Perform three sets of 10-12 reps. Select a different exercise for each training day.

Beginner Program

Day 3 (Optional – For Physique-focused Clients)

A1) Bicep Curl (BB)	Sets x Reps	Intensity	Rest
Week 1	5x 10	★	60s
Week 2	6 x 10	★	60s
Week 3	8 x 10	★	60s
Week 4	10 x 10	★	60s

Note: use a weight you are comfortable with for 15 repetitions. If you are able to complete all sets for 10 repetitions, increase the weight on the bar by 5%.

A2) Tricep Extension (BB)	Sets x Reps	Intensity	Rest
Week 1	5 x 10	★	60s
Week 2	6 x 10	★	60s
Week 3	8 x 10	★	60s
Week 4	10 x 10	★	60s

Note: use a weight you are comfortable with for 15 repetitions. If you are able to complete all sets for 10 repetitions, increase the weight on the bar by 5%.

B1) Supplementary Exercise	Reps	Rest
Choose one exercise from LIST A	3 x 10-12	0s

B2) Supplementary Exercise	Reps	Rest
Choose one exercise from LIST B	3 x 10-12	0s

Choose from the supplementary exercises shown in List A and List B on page 242. Perform three sets of 10-12 reps. Select a different exercise for each training day.

BEGINNER CARDIO (HIIT) – *See Appendix B*

Moderate/Advanced Program: Strength Training
Day 1 (Deadlift/Push – Monday)

Exercise	Reps	Rest
A1) Deadlifts	10 x 10	60s
B1) Bench Press	10 x 10	60s
C1) Supplementary Exercise – List A	3 x 10-12	0s
C2) Supplementary Exercise – List B	3 x 10-12	0s

Note: Use a weight you are comfortable with for 12 repetitions. If you are able to complete all sets for 10 repetitions, increase the weight on the bar by 10lb for lower body exercises and 5lb for upper body exercises.

Day 2 (Squat/Pull – Thursday)

Exercise	Reps	Rest
A1) Back Squats	10 x 10	60s
B1) Chin-Ups (use bodyweight)	10 x 10	60s
C1) Supplementary Exercise – List A	3 x 10-12	-
C2) Supplementary Exercise – List B	3 x 10-12	-

Note: Use a weight you are comfortable with for 12 repetitions. If you are able to complete all sets for 10 repetitions, increase the weight on the bar by 10lb for lower body exercises and 5lb for upper body exercises.

Day 3 (Arms – Optional, For Physique-focused Clients]

Exercise	Reps	Rest
A1) Barbell Drag Curl	10 x 10	60s
B1) Narrow-Grip Dips	10 x 10	60s
C1) Supplementary Exercise – List A	3 x 10-12	0s
C2) Supplementary Exercise – List B	3 x 10-12	0s

Note: Use a weight you are comfortable with for 12 repetitions. If you are able to complete all sets for 10 repetitions, increase the weight on the bar by 5lb for upper-body exercises.

Weekly Progression For Moderate/Advanced Program

Week 1 – 70% of 1RM

Week 2 – 70% of 1RM (Perform more total reps than Week 1)

Week 3 – 70% of 1RM (Perform more total reps than Week 2)

Week 4 – 70% of 1RM (Perform more total reps than Week 3)

Note: If you are able to complete all sets for 10 repetitions, increase the weight on the bar by 10% (lower-body exercises) and 5% (upper-body exercises)

Moderate/Advanced Program: Cardio (HIIT)

– See Appendix E

APPENDIX E

HIIT FOR PERFORMANCE

Perform HIIT sprints twice weekly for four to eight weeks, then evaluate progress and re-assess.

Phase I

WEEK	WORKOUT (Sets x Distance)	REST PERIOD
1	8 x 100m	60s
2	10 x 100m	60s
3	12 x 100m	60s
4	15 x 100m	60s

Phase II

WEEK	WORKOUT (Sets x Distance)	REST PERIOD
5	5 x 200m	120s
6	6 x 200m	120s
7	7 x 200m	120s
8	8 x 200m	120s

REFERENCES

Chapter 1

1. Koopmen R et al. Combined ingestion of protein and free leucine with carbohydrate increases post-exercise muscle protein synthesis in vivo male subjects. Am J Physiol Endocrinol Metab 2005;288(5):E645-E653.

2. Kim D, et al. mTOR interacts with raptor to form a nutrient-sensitive complex that signals to the cell growth machinery. Cell 2002, 110:163–175.

3. Xu G et al. Metabolic regulation by leucine and translation initiation through the mTOR-signalling pathway by pancreatic B-cells. Diabetes 2001;50:353-360.

4. Layman DK, BAUM JI. Dietary protein impact on glycemic control during weight loss. J Nutr 2004;134(4):968S-973S.

5. Adapted from http://www.elmhurst.edu/~chm/vchembook/600glycolysis.html

6. Schaafsma, Gertjan. PDCAAS, protein digestibility–corrected amino acid score. J. Nutr. July 1, 2000 vol. 130 no. 7 1865S-1867S.

7. Lowery LM, Devia L. Dietary protein safety and resistance exercise: what do we really know? J Int Soc Sports Nutr. 2009 Jan 12;6:3.

8. Zavorsky G, et al. An open-label dose-response study of lymphocyte glutathione levels in healthy men and women receiving pressurized whey protein isolate supplements. Int J Food Sci Nutr. 2007 Sep;58(6):429-36.

9. J Nutr. 2002 Aug;132(8):2174-8. Pal, S. Ellis, V. The chronic effects of whey proteins on blood pressure, vascular function, and inflammatory markers in overweight individuals. Obesity (Silver Springs) 2010 Jul;18(7):1354-9.

10. Phillips SM. The science of muscle hypertrophy: making dietary protein count. Proc Nutr Soc. 2011 Feb;70(1):100-3.

11. Calbet JA, MacLean DA. Plasma glucagon and insulin responses depend on the rate of appearance of amino acids after ingestion of different protein solutions in humans. J Nutr. 2002 Aug;132(8):2174-82.

12. Stark M et al. Protein timing and its effects on muscular hypertrophy and strength in individuals engaged in weight-training. J Int Sports Nutr. 2012 Dec 14;9(1):54.

13. Blomstrand E, Saltin B. Effect of muscle glycogen on glucose, lactate and amino acid metabolism during exercise and recovery in human subjects. J Physiol. 1999 Jan 1; 514 (Pt 1) :293-302.

14. Cribb PJ, Hayes A. Effects of supplement timing and resistance exercise on skeletal muscle hypertrophy. Med Sci Sport Exerc. 2006 Nov;38(11):1918-25.

15. Gardner C et al. Comparison of the Atkins, Zone, Ornish, and LEARN diets for change in weight and related risk factors among overweight premenopausal women: the A TO Z Weight Loss Study: a randomized trial. *JAMA*. 2007;297(9):969-977.

16. Weigle D et al. Am J Clin Nutr. 2005 Jul;82(1):41-8.A high-protein diet induces sustained reductions in appetite, ad libitum caloric intake, and body weight despite compensatory changes in diurnal plasma leptin and ghrelin concentrations.

17. Wycherley T et al. Am J Clin Nutr. 2012 Dec;96(6):1281-98. doi: 10.3945/ajcn.112.044321. Epub 2012 Oct 24. Effects of energy-restricted high-protein, low-fat compared with standard-protein, low-fat diets: a meta-analysis of randomized controlled trials.

18. Clifton P et al. High protein diets decrease total and abdominal fat and improve CVD risk profile in overweight and obese men and women with elevated triacylglycerol. Nutr Metab Cardiovasc Dis. 2009 Oct;19(8):548-54.

19. Appel LJ, et al; the OmniHeart Collaborative Research Group. Effects of protein, monounsaturated fat, and carbohydrate intake on blood pressure and serum lipids: results of the OmniHeart randomized trial. JAMA. 2005;294:2455-2464.

20. Santesso N et al. Effects of higher- versus lower-protein diets on health outcomes: a systematic review and meta-analysis. Eur J Clin Nutr. 2012 Jul;66(7):780-8.

21.	Hu, F. Protein, body weight, and cardiovascular health. Am J Clin Nutr, 2005 Jul;82(1 Suppl):242S-247S.

22.	Pannomans DL et al 1997 'Calcium excretion, apparent calcium absoption and calcium balance inyoung and elderly subjects:influence of protein intake.' Brit J Nutr, Vol 77(5), pp.721-9.

23.	Antonio, J et al. Essentials of Sports Nutrition and Supplements. Humana Press. New York, NY.

24.	http://www.precisionnutrition.com/calorie-control-guide

Chapter 2

1.	Erasmus, Udo. Fats That Heal & Fats That Kill. Alive Books. Burnaby, BC. 1993

2.	Siri-Tarino PW, et al. Meta-analysis of prospective cohort studies evaluating the association of saturated fat with cardiovascular disease Am J Clin Nutr 13 January 2010

3.	Geng Z. et al. Associations of erythrocyte palmitoleic acid with adipokines, inflammatory markers, and the metabolic syndrome in middle-aged and older Chinese Am J Clin Nutr. 2012 November; 96(5): 970–976.

4.	Okada, Y et al. Trans fatty acids in diets act as a precipitating factor for gut inflammation? J Gastroenterol Hepatol 2013 Dec;28 Suppl 4:29-32.

5.	Surette, M et al. Inhibition of leukotriene biosynthesis by a novel dietary fatty acid formulation in patients with atopic asthma: a randomized, placebo-controlled, parallel-group, prospective trial. Clin Ther. 2003 Mar;25(3):972-9.

6.	Levanthal, L et al. Treatment of rheumatoid arthritis with gammalinolenic acid. Ann Intern Med. 1993 Nov 1;119(9):867-73.

7.	Kawamura, A et al. Dietary supplementation of gamma-linolenic acid improves skin parameters in subjects with dry skin and mild atopic dermatitis. J Oleo Sci. 2011;60(12):597-607.

8.	Serhan C, Petasis N. Resolvins and protectins in inflammation resolution. Chem Rev. 2011 Oct 12;111(10):5922-43.

9.	Mozaffarian D, Lemaitre RN, King IB, et al. Plasma phospholipid long-chain omega-3 fatty acids and total and cause-specific mortality in older adults. A cohort study. Ann Intern Med 2013; 158:515-525.

10. Smith GI et al. Omega-3 polyunsaturated fatty acids augment the muscle protein anabolic response to hyperinsulinaemia-hyperaminoacidaemia in healthy young and middle-aged men and women. Clin Sci (Lond). 2011 Sep;121(6):267-78

11. Adapted
from http://www.elmhurst.edu/~chm/vchembook/600glycolysis.html

12. Assuncao ML et al. Effects of dietary coconut oil on the biochemical and anthropometric profiles of women presenting abdominal obesity. Lipids. 2009 Jul;44(7):593-60.

13. Takeuchi H et al. The application of medium-chain fatty acids: edible oil with a suppressing effect on body fat accumulation. Asia Pac J Clin Nutr 2008;17 Suppl 1:320-3.

14. Smit LA et al Conjugated linoleic acid in adipose tissue and risk of myocardial infarction. 2010 Jul;92(1):34-40.

15. Burdge GC, Jones AE, Wootton SA. Eicosapentaenoic and docosapentaenoic acids are the principal products of alpha-linolenic acid metabolism in young men*. Br J Nutr. 2002;88(4):355-364.

16. Burdge GC, Wootton SA. Conversion of alpha-linolenic acid to eicosapentaenoic, docosapentaenoic and docosahexaenoic acids in young women. Br J Nutr. 2002;88(4):411-420.

17. Manerba A, Vizzardi E, Metra M, Dei Cas L (2010) n-3 PUFAs and cardiovascular disease prevention. Future Cardiol 6:343–350

18. Meyer BJ, Lane AE, Mann NJ (2009) Comparison of seal oil to tuna oil on plasma lipid levels and blood pressure in hypertri- glyceridaemic subjects. Lipids 44:827–835

19. Cordain L. The Paleo Diet. John Wiley & Sons. New Jersey, 2002

20. Hibbeln, JR et al. "Healthy intakes of n−3 and n−6 fatty acids: estimations considering worldwide diversity". American Journal of Clinical Nutrition. June 1, 2006. 83 (6, supplement): 1483S–1493S.

21. Okuyama, H et al. "ω3 fatty acids effectively prevent coronary heart disease and other late-onset diseases: the excessive linoleic acid syndrome". World Review of Nutritional Dietetics. World Review of Nutrition and Dietetics (Karger) 2007, 96 (Prevention of Coronary Heart Disease): 83–103.

22. Cordain, L. OAND Convention 2013. Origin and Evolution of the Western diet: Health Implications for the 21st century. (Lecture) Nov 16th, 2013. Toronto, ON.

23. Volek J et al. Testosterone and cortisol in relationship to dietary nutrients and resistance exercise. Osteoarthritis Cartilage. 2009 Jul;17(7):896-905.

24. Phillips T et al. A dietary supplement attenuates IL-6 and CRP after eccentric exercise in untrained males. Med Sci Sports Exerc 2003;35(12):2032-2037

25. Nosaka N et al. Effect of ingestion of medium-chain triacylglycerols on moderate- and high-intensity exercise in recreational athletes. J Nutr Sci Vitaminol (Tokyo) 2009 Apr;55(2):120-5.

26. Delarue J et al. Fish oil attenuates adrenergic overactivity without altering glucose metabolism during an oral glucose load in haemodialysis patients. Br J Nutr. 2008 May;99(5):1041-7.

27. Hellhammer J et al. Omega-3 fatty acids administered in phosphatidyl-serine improved certain aspects of high chronic stress in men. Nutr Res. 2012 Apr;32(4):241-50.

28. Delarue J et al. Interaction of fish oil and a glucocorticoid on metabolic responses to an oral glucose load in healthy human subjects. Br J Nutr. 2006 Feb;95(2):267-72.

29. Dorgan JF. Effects of dietary fat and fiber on plasma and urine androgens and estrogens in men: a controlled feeding study. Am J Clin Nutr. 1996 Dec;64(6):850-5.

30. Zainal, Z et al. Relative efficacies of omega-3 polyunsaturated fatty acids in reducing expression of key proteins in a model system for studying osteoarthritis. Osteoarthritis Cartilage. 2009 Jul;17(7):896-905.

31. Siriwardhana N et al. Health benefits of n-3 polyunsaturated fatty acids: eicosapentaenoic acid and docosahexaenoic acid. Adv Food Nutr Res. 2012;65:211-22.

32. Su K, Huang S, Chiu C, Shen W. Omega-3 fatty acids in major depressive disorder. A preliminary double-blind, placebo-controlled trial. Eur Neuropsychopharmacol 2003;13(4):267-271

33. Martins JG. EPA but not DHA appears to be responsible for the efficacy of omega-3 long chain polyunsaturated fatty acid supplementation in depression: evidence from a meta-analysis of randomized controlled trials. J Am Coll Nutr. 2009 Oct;28(5):525-42.

Chapter 3

1. Gallop R. The G.I. Diet – Glycemic Index. Workman Publishing 2010.

2. Cordain L. The Paleo Diet. John Wiley & Sons. New Jersey, 2002

3. Anderson JW. Whole grains and coronary heart disease: the whole kernel of truth. Am J Clin Nutr. 2004 Dec;80(6):1459-60. 2004.

4. Pusztai A. Dietary lectins are metabolic signals for the gut and modulate immune and hormone functions. Eur J Clin Nutr 1993 Oct;47(10):691-9.

5. Bueno, N et al. Very-low-carbohydrate ketogenic diet v. low-fat diet for long-term weight loss: a meta-analysis of randomised controlled trials. Br J Nutr. 2013 Oct;110(7):1178-87.

6. Perez-Guisado, J. Munoz-Serrano A. A pilot study of the Spanish Ketogenic Mediterranean Diet: an effective therapy for the metabolic syndrome. J Med Food. 2011 Jul-Aug;14(7-8):681-7.

7. Ballard, K et al. Dietary carbohydrate restriction improves insulin sensitivity, blood pressure, microvascular function, and cellular adhesion markers in individuals taking statins. Nutr Res. 2013 Nov;33(11):905-12.

8. Crane P. et al. Glucose Levels and Risk of Dementia. NEJM. Sept 2013 Vol 369.

9. Ivy JL et al. Muscle glycogen storage after different amounts of carbohydrate ingestion. J Appl Physiol. 1988 Nov;65(5):2018-23

10. Wong SH et al. Effect of glycemic index meals on recovery and subsequent endurance capacity. Int J Sports Med. 2009 Dec;30(12):898-905.

11. Tappy L, Le KA. Metabolic effects of fructose and the worldwide increase in obesity. Physiol Rev. 2010 Jan;90(1):23-46.

12. Payne AN et al. Gut microbial adaptation to dietary consumption of fructose, artificial sweeteners and sugar alcohols: implications for host-microbe interactions contributing to obesity. Obes Rev. 2012 Sep;13(9):799-809.

13. de Koning L, Malik VS, Kellogg MD et al. Sweetened beverage consumption, incident coronary heart disease and biomarkers of risk in men. Circulation 2012

14. Center for Disease Control and Prevention MMWR Weekly. 2012;61

15. http://www.precisionnutrition.com/calorie-control-guide

Chapter 4

1. Leischeid, D. OAND Conference Lecture. 2008 volume 5. Audio recording

2. Pizzorno J, Murray MT. Textbook of Natural Medicine. New York, NY. Churchill Livingstone, 1999:245-46.

3. Guyton, A. Hall, J. Textbook of Medical Physiology, 10th Ed. Guyton Physiology. 2010

4. Wright, J. Why Stomach Acid Is Good for You: Natural Relief from Heartburn, Indigestion, Reflux and GERD.

5. Robillard, N. Fast Track Digestion Heartburn (Ebook) Oct, 2012.

6. Prousky, J. Principles & Practices of Naturopathic Clinical Nutrition. 2008. CCNM Press.

7. Thorens J et al. Bacterial overgrowth during treatment with omeprazole compared with cimetidine: a prospective. Gut. 1996 Jul;39(1):54-9.

8. Marsh MN, Crowe PT. Morphology of the mucosal lesion in gluten sensitivity. Baillieres Clin Gastroenterol. 1995 Jun;9(2):273-93.

9. Hawrelak J, Myers S. The causes of intestinal dysbiosis: review. Alt Med Rev 2004;9:180-97.

10. http://www.who.int/drugresistance/WHO_Global_Strategy_English.pdf. WHO Global Strategy for Containment of Antimicrobial Resistance.

11. Kane, M, Saputo, L. Boosting Your Digestive Health. Octopus Publising NY, 2002.

12. Miller AL. The pathogenesis, clinical implications, and treatment of intestinal hyperpermeability. Altern Med Rev 1997;2:330-45.

13. Bjarnason I et al. Review Side effects of nonsteroidal anti-inflammatory drugs on the small and large intestine in humans. Gastroenterology. 1993 Jun; 104(6):1832-47.

14. Maiden L et al. Long-term effects of nonsteroidal anti-inflammatory drugs and cyclooxygenase-2 selective agents on the small bowel: a cross-sectional capsule enteroscopy study. Clin Gastroenterol Hepatol. 2007 Sep; 5(9):1040-5. Epub 2007 Jul 10.

15. Matsui H et al. The pathophysiology of non-steroidal anti-inflammatory drug (NSAID)-induced mucosal injuries in stomach and small intestine. J Clin Biochem Nutr. 2011 Mar;48(2):107-11

16. Titgemeyer EC, Bourquin LD, Fahey GC Jr, et al. Fermentability of various fiber sources by human fecal bacteria in vitro. Am J Clin Nutr 1991;53(6):1418-24

17. Estruch R et al. Effects of dietary fibre intake on risk factors for cardiovascular disease in subjects at high risk. J Epidemiol Community Health. 2009 Jul;63(7):582-8

18. Ringel-Kulta T et al. Probiotic bacteria Lactobacillus acidophilus NCFM and Bifidobacterium lactis Bi-07 versus placebo for the symptoms of bloating in patients with functional bowel disorders: a double-blind study. J Clin Gastroenterol. 2011 Jul 45(6):518-25

19. Yang YJ et al..Lactobacillus acidophilus ameliorates H. pylori-induced gastric inflammation by inactivating the Smad7 and NFκB pathways. BMC Mibrobiol. 2012 Mar 19;12:38

20. Lee JS et al. Anti-inflammatory actions of probiotics through activating suppressor of cytokine signaling (SOCS) expression and signaling in Helicobacter pylori infection: a novel mechanism. J Gastroenterol Hepatol. 2010 Jan;25(1):194-202

21. Sabater-Molina M et al. Dietary fructooligosaccharides and potential benefits on health. J Physiol Biochem. 2009 Sep;65(3):315-28

22. Liu, Y., et al. "Update on berberine in nonalcoholic Fatty liver disease". Evidence-Based Complementary and Alternative Medicine Vol. 2013 (2013): 308134.

23. Vermeulen MA et al. Glutamate reduces experimental intestinal hyperpermeability and facilitates glutamine support of gut integrity. World J Gastroenterol. 2011 Mar 28;17(12):1569-73

24. Antonio, J et al. Essentials of Sports Nutrition and Supplements. Humana Press. New York, NY.

25. Lastra C et al. Antiucler and gastroprotective effects of quercetin: a gross and histologic study. Pharmacology 1994; 48:56-62 Skaper S et al.

26. Quercetin protects cutaneous tissue associated cell types including sensory neurons from oxidative stress induced by glutathione depletion: cooperative effects of ascorbic acid. Fr Rad Biol Med 1997;22(4):669

27. Crowe S, Perdue M. Functional abnormalities in the intestine associated with mucosal mast cell activation. Reg Immunol 1992;4:113-17.

28.   Sturniolo GC et al. Zinc supplementation tightens "leaky gut" in Crohn's disease. Inflamm Bowel Dis. 2001 May; 7(2):94-8

Chapter 5

1.   Rask C et al. Differential effect on cell-mediated immunity in human volunteers after intake of different lactobacilli. Clin Exp Immunol 2013 May;172(2):321-32.

2.   Purchiaroni F et al. The role of intestinal microbiota and the immune system. Eur Rev Med Pharmacol Sci 2013 Feb;17(3):323-33.

3.   Pender, M. CD8+ T-Cell Deficiency, Epstein-Barr Virus Infection, Vitamin D Deficiency, andSteps to Autoimmunity: A Unifying Hypothesis. Autoimmune Dis 2012;2012:189096.

4.   Urashima M, et al. Randomized trial of vitamin D supplementation to prevent seasonal influenza A in schoolchildren. Am J Clin Nutr. 2010 May;91(5):1255-60.

5.   http://www.vitamindsociety.org/

6.   Semba RD. The role of vitamin A and related retinoids in immune function. Nutr Rev. 1998;56(1 Pt 2):S38-48

7.   McCullough, F. et al. The effect of vitamin A on epithelial integrity. Nutr Soc. 1999; volume 58: pages 289-293

8.   Douglas RM et al. Vitamin C for preventing and treating the common cold. Cochrane Database Systematic Review. 2004 Oct 18;(4):CD000980.

9.   Peters EM, Goetzche JM, Grobbelaar B, Noakes TD. Vitamin C supplementation reduces the incidence of post race symptoms of upper-respiratory-tract infection in ultra marathon runners. Am J Clin Nutr 1993 Feb;57(2):170-4.

10.   Mangini S et al. A combination of high-dose vitamin C plus zinc for the common cold. J Int Med Res. 2012;40(1):28-42.

11.   Konig D, Weinstock C, Keul J, Northoff H, Berg A. Zinc, iron, and magnesium status in athletes: influence on the reuglation of exercise-induced stress and immune function. Exerc Immunol Rev 1998;4:2-21.

12.   Castell LM, Newsholme EA. The effects of oral glutamine supplementation on athletes after prolonged, exhaustive exercise. Nutrition. 1997 Jul-Aug;13(7-8):738-42.

13. Kim H. Glutamine as an immunonutrient. Yonsei Med J. 2011 Nov;52(6):892-97

14. Antonio, J et al. Essentials of Sports Nutrition and Supplements. Humana Press. New York, NY.

15. Madden J.A.J. et al. Effect of probiotics on preventing disruption of the intestinal microflora following antibiotic therapy: A double-blind, placebo-controlled pilot study. Int Immunophar 2005: 5: 1091-1097.

16. Susan F. Plummer et al. Effects of probiotics on the composition of the intestinal microbiota following antibiotic therapy. International Journal of Antimicrobial Agents 2005: 26: 69-74.

17. Novas AM et al. Tennis, incidence of URTI and salivary IgA. Int J Sports Med. 2003 Apr;24(3):223-9

18. Kakanis et al. The open window of susceptibility to infection after acute exercise in healthy young male elite athletes Exerc Immunol Rev 2010;16:119-37

19. Walsh PH et al. Position statement. Part one: Immune function and exercise. Exerc Immunol Rev. 2011;17:6-63. 3

20. Tsai et al. Resting salivary levels of IgA and cortisol are significantly affected during intensive resistance training periods in elite male weightlifters.J Strength Cond Res. 2012 Aug;26(8):2202-8

21. He CS et al. Relationships among salivary immunoglobulin A, lactoferrin and cortisol in basketball players during a basketball season. Eur J Appl Physiol. 2010 Nov;110(5):989-95

22. Suzui M et al. Natural killer cell lytic activity and CD56(dim) and CD56(bright) cell distributions during and after intensive training. J Appl Physiol. 2004 Jun;96(6):2167-73.

23. Rystedt LW et al. Long-term impact of role stress and cognitive rumination upon morning and evening saliva cortisol secretion. Ergonomics 2011 May;54(5):430-5.

24. Rystedt LW et al. The relationship between long-term job strain and morning and evening saliva cortisol secretion among white-collar workers. J Occup Health Psychol. 2008 Apr;13(2):105-13.

25. Fondell E et al. Short natural sleep is associated with higher T cell and lower NK cell activities.Brain Behav Immun. 2011 Oct;25(7):1367-75.

26. Schwellnus M., Lichaba M., Derman E. Respiratory tract symptoms in endurance athletes—A review of causes and consequences. Curr. Allergy Clin. Immunol. 2010;23:52–57.

27. Nieman, D et al. Upper respiratory tract infection is reduced in physically fit and active adults. Br J Sports Med. 2011 Sep;45(12):987-92

28. Shao, B.M., et al. "A study on the immune receptors for polysaccharides from the roots of Astragalus membranaceus, a Chinese medicinal herb". Biochemical and Biophysical Research Communications 320, No. 4 (2004): 1103–1111.

29. Bernardes de Jesus, M et al. The telomerase activator TA-65 elongates short telomeres and increases health span of adult/old mice without increasing cancer incidence. Aging Cell 2011 Aug;10(4):604-21.

30. Kodama N et al. Effect of Maitake (Grifola frondosa) D-Fraction on the activation of NK cells in cancer patients. J Med Food. 2003 Winter;6(4):371-7.

31. Ike K et al. Induction of a T-Helper 1 (Th1) immune response in mice by an extract from the Pleurotus eryngii (Eringi) mushroom. J Med Food.2012 Dec;15(12):1124-8. doi: 10.1089/jmf.2012.2239.

32. Davison G, Diment BC. Bovine colostrum supplementation attenuates the decrease of salivary lysozyme and enhances the recovery of neutrophil function after prolonged exercise. Br J Nutr 2010 May;103(10):1425-32.

33. Cao J, Zhang Y, Chen W, Zhao X. The relationship between fasting plasma concentrations of selected flavonoids and their ordinary dietary intake. Br J Nutr 2010;103:249-255

34. Kelly, G. Quercetin: Monograph. Alternative Med Review.Vol 16; No 2.

35. Liu Y et al. 'Update on berberine in nonalcoholic fatty liver disease.' Evidence-based complementary and alternative medicine. Vol. 2013 (2013): 308134.

Chapter 6

1. Emerging Risk Factors Collaboration. Diabetes mellitus, fasting glucose, and risk of cause-specific death. New England Journal Medicine, Mar 2011;364;9:328-341.

2. G. S. Hotamisligil, N. S. Shargill, and B. M. Spiegelman, "Adipose expression of tumor necrosis factor-α: direct role in obesity-linked insulin resistance," Science, vol. 259, no. 5091, pp. 87–91, 1993.

3.   S. E. Wozniak, L. L. Gee, M. S. Wachtel, and E. E. Frezza, "Adipose tissue: the new endocrine organ? a review article," Digestive Diseases and Sciences, vol. 54, no. 9, pp. 1847–1856, 2009.

4.   Chearskul S et al. Obesity and appetite-related hormones. J Med Assoc Thai. 2012 Nov;95(11):1472-9.

5.   Beccuti G, Pannain S. Sleep and obesity. Curr Opin Clin Nutr Metab Care. 2011 Jul;14(4):402-12.

6.   Lee KY et al. Exercise improves adiponectin concentrations irrespective of the adiponectin gene polymorphisms SNP45 and the SNP276 in obese Korean women. Gene. 2013 Mar 10;516(2):271-6. doi: 10.1016/j. gene.2012.12.028. Epub 2012 Dec 28.

7.   S. Gesta, Y.-H. Tseng, and C. R. Kahn, "Developmental origin of fat: tracking obesity to its source," Cell, vol. 131, no. 2, pp. 242–256, 2007.

8.   R. Cancello and K. Clément, "Is obesity an inflammatory illness? Role of low-grade inflammation and macrophage infiltration in human white adipose tissue," International Journal of Obstetrics & Gynaecology, vol. 113, no. 10, pp. 1141–1147, 2006

9.   Richard D et al. Determinants of brown adipocyte development and thermogenesis. Int J Obes (Lond). 2010 Dec;34 Suppl 2:s59-66. doi: 10.1038/ijo.2010.241.

10.   Drago S et al. Gliadin, zonulin and gut permeability: Effects on celiac and non-celiac intestinal mucosa and intestinal cell lines. Scand J Gastroenterol. 2006 Apr;41(4):408-19.

11.   Fasano A. Zonulin and its regulation of intestinal barrier function: the biological door to inflammation, autoimmunity, and cancer. Physiol Rev 2011 Jan;91(1):151-75.

12.   Moreno-Navarrete JM et al. Circulating zonulin, a marker of intestinal permeability, is increased in association with obesity-associated insulin resistance. PLos One 2012;7(5):e37160.

13.   VanWijck K et al. Aggravation of exercise-induced intestinal injury by Ibroprofen in athletes. Med Sci Sports Exerc. 2012 Dec;44(12):2257-62.

14.   Matsui H et al. The pathophysiology of non-steroidal anti-inflammatory drug (NSAID)-induced mucosal injuries in stomach and small intestine. J Clin Biochem Nutr. 2011 Mar;48(2):107-11

15.   Pederson B et al. Exercise-induced immunodulation: possible roles of neu-
roendocrine and metabolic forces. Int J Spors Med 1997;18(Suppl 1):S2-7

16.   Buyken AE et al. Carbohydrate nutrition and inflammatory disease mortality
in older adults. Am J Clin Nutr.2010;92(3):634-43.

17.   Harris TB et al. Associations of elevated interleukin-6 and C-reactive protein
levels with mortality in the elderly. Am J Med. 1999 May; 106(5):506-12

18.   Phillips T et al. A dietary supplement attenuates IL=6 ad CRP after eccentric
exercise in untrained males. Med Sci Sports Exerc 2003;35(12):2032-2037

19.   Rangel-Huerta OD, Aguilera CM, Mesa MD, Gil A.   Br J Nutr. 2012
Jun;107 Suppl 2:S159-70. Omega-3 long-chain polyunsaturated fatty acids
supplementation on inflammatory biomakers: a systematic review of randomised clinical trials.

20.   Nakachi K et al. Preventive effects of drinking green tea on cancer and cardiovascular disease: epidemiological evidence for multiple targeting prevention. : Biofactors 2000;13(1 - 4):49 - 54.

21.   Masuda Y et al. Antioxidant properties of gingerol related compounds from
ginger. Biofactors. 2004;21(104):293-296

22.   Dugasi S, et al. Comparative antioxidant and anti-inflammatory
effects of [6]-gingerol, [8]-gingerol, [10]-gingerol and [6]-shogaol. J
Ethnopharmacol. 2010;127(2):515-520.

23.   Percival SS et al. Bioavailability of herbs and spices in humans as determined
by ex vivo inflammatory suppression and DNA strand breaks. J Am Coll
Nutr. 2012 Aug;31(4):288-94.

24.   Liu Y, Nair MG. Capsaicinoids in the hottest pepper Bhut Jolokia and
its antioxidant and anti-inflammatory activities. Nat Prod Commun
2010 Jan;5(1):91-94

25.   Rao, TS, et al. Anti-inflammatory activity of curcumin analogues. Ind J.Med.
Res.,1982. 75:574 – 578

26.   De la Lastra C, Villegas I. Resveratrol as an anti-inflammatory and anti-
aging agent; mechanism and clinical implications. Mol Nutr Food Res.
2005 May;49(5):405-430.

27.   Zahedi HS et al. Effects of polygonum cuspidatum containing resveratrol
on inflammation in male professional basketball players. Int J Prev Med.
2013 Apr;4(Supppl1):S1-4.

28. Crandall JP et al. Pilot study of resveratrol in older adults with impaired glucose tolerance. J Gerontol A Biol Sci Med Sci. 2012 Dec;67(12):1307-12

29. Timmers S et al. Therapeutic potential of resveratrol in obesity and type 2 diabetes: new avenues for health benefits. Ann NY Acad Sci. 2013 Jul;1290(1):83-9. doi: 10.1111/nyas.12185.

Chapter 7

1. Antonio, J et al. Essentials of Sports Nutrition and Supplements. Humana Press. New York, NY.

2. Houmard JA et al. Seven days of exercise increase GLUT-4 protein content in human skeletal muscle. J Appl Physiol 1995 Dec;79(6):1936-8.

3. Stark M et al. Protein timing and its effects on muscular hypertrophy and strength in individuals engaged in weight-training. J Int Sports Nutr. 2012 Dec 14;9(1):54.

4. Ginter E, Simko V. Type 2 diabetes mellitus, pandemic in 21st century. Adv Exp Med Biol. 2012;771:42-50

5. Taubes, G. Is Sugar Toxic? New York Times, April 13, 2011

6. Payne AN et al. Gut microbial adaptation to dietary consumption of fructose, artificial sweeteners and sugar alcohols: implications for host-microbe interactions contributing to obesity. Obes Rev. 2012 Sep;13(9):799-809.

7. Sievenpiper, J et al. Effect of Fructose on Body Weight in Controlled Feeding Trials: A Systematic Review and Meta-analysis. Ann Intern Med. 2012;156(4):291-304.

8. Brennan IM et al. Effects of fat, protein, and carbohydrate and protein load on appetite, plasma cholecystokinin, peptide YY, and ghrelin, and energy intake in lean and obese men. Am J Physiol Gastrointest Liver Phsyiol 2012 Jul;303(1):G129-40.

9. Malaisse WJ et al. Effects of artificial sweeteners on insulin release and cationic fluxes in rat pancreatic islets. Cell Signal. 1998 Nov;10(10):727-33.

10. Wiklund AK, et al. Sucralose - an ecotoxicological challenger? Chemoshpere 2012 Jan;86(1):50-5.

11. Karstadt ML. Inadequate Toxicity tests of food additive. 2010 Jan-mar;(16(1):89-96

12. Nutt D, King LA, Saulsbury W, Blakemore C (2007) Development of a rational scale to assess the harm of drugs of potential misuse. Lancet 369: 1047–1053

13. Lenoir M et al. Intense Sweetness Surpasses Cocaine Reward. Plus One 2007 Aug 1;2(8):e698.

14. Misra M et al. Increased carbohydrate induced ghrelin secretion in obese vs. normal-weight adolescent girls. Obesity. 2009 Sep;17(9):1689-95.

15. Schmid S et al. A single night of sleep deprivation increases ghrelin levels and feelings of hunger in normal-weight healthy men. J Sleep Res. 2008 Sep;17(3):331-4.

16. Timonen. M et al. Insulin resistance and depressive symptoms in young adult males: Findings from Finnish military conscripts. Psychosom Med 69(8):723-28.

17. Pyykkonen AJ et al. Depressive symptoms, antidepressant medication use, and insulin resistance: the PPP-Botnia Study. Diabetes Care. 2011 Dec;34(12):2545-7.

18. Pagana K, Pagana T. Manual of Diagnostic and Laboratory Tests 2nd Ed. Mosby's Publ. 2002

19. Jonsson T, Beneficial effects of a Paleolithic diet on cardiovascular risk factors in type-2 diabetes:a randomized cross-over pilot study. 2009 Jul 16;8:35

20. Selvin. Meta-analysis: glycosylated hemoglobin and cardiovascular disease in diabetes mellitus. Ann Intern Med. 2004;141:421-31

21. Lindeberg S et al. A Palaeolithic diet improves glucose tolerance more than a Mediterranean-like diet in individuals with ischaemic heart disease. Diabetologia. 2007;50(9):1795–807.

22. Frasetto LA. Metabolic and physiologic improvements from consuming a paleolithic, hunter-gatherer type diet. Eur J Clin Nutr 2009 Aug;63(8):947-55.

23. Mavros Y et al. Changes in Insulin Resistance and HbA1c Are Related to Exercise-Mediated Changes in Body Composition in Older Adults With Type 2 Diabetes. Diabetes Care. March 8th, 2013

24. Gillen GB, et al. Acute high-intensity interval exercise reduces the postprandial glucose response and prevalence of hyperglycaemia in patients with type 2 diabetes. 2012 Jun;14(6):575-7.

25. Khan, et al. Cinnamon improves glucose and lipids of people with type 2 diabetes. Diabetes Care. 2003; 26:3215-18

26. Davis PA and Yokoyama W. Cinnamon intake lowers fasting blood glucose: meta-analysis. J Med Food. 2011 Sep;14(9):884-9. doi: 10.1089/jmf.2010.0180.

27. Lu T et al. Cinnamon extract improves fasting blood glucose and glycosylated hemoglobin level in Chinese patients with type 2 diabetes. Nutr Res 2012 Jun;32(6):408-12.

28. Poh ZX, Goh KO. A current update on the use of alpha lipoic acid in the management of type 2 diabetes mellitus. Endocr Metab Immune Disord Drug Targets. 2009 Dec;9(4):392-8.

29. Zhang et al. Amelioration of lipid abnormalities by α-lipoic acid through antioxidative and anti-inflammatory effects. Obesity (Silver Springs) 2011 Aug;19(8):1647-53.

30. Harding SV et al. J Diet Suppl 2012 Jun;9(2):116-27. Evidence for using alpha-lipoic acid in reducing lipoprotein and inflammatory related atherosclerotic risk.

31. Khabbazzi T et al. Effects of alpha-lipoic acid supplementation on inflammation, oxidative stress, and serum lipid profile levels in patients with end-stage renal disease on hemodialysis. J Ren Nutr 2012 Mar;22(2):244-50.

32. Yin, J., H. Xing, and J. Ye. "Efficacy of berberine in patients with type 2 diabetes mellitus". Metabolism Vol. 57, No. 5 (2008): 712–717.

33. Zhang, H., et al. "Berberine lowers blood glucose in type 2 diabetes mellitus patients through increasing insulin receptor expression". Metabolism Vol. 59, No. 2 (2010): 285–292

34. Han, J., H. Lin, and W. Huang. "Modulating gut microbiota as an antidiabetic mechanism of berberine". Medical Science Monitor Vol. 17, No. 7 (2011): RA164–RA167.

35. Liu, Y., et al. "Update on berberine in nonalcoholic Fatty liver disease". Evidence-Based Complementary and Alternative Medicine Vol. 2013 (2013): 308134.

Chapter 8

1. Reynolds G. The Hormone Edge. J of Physio. NY Jan 14, 2012.

2. Thaler J et al. Obesity-induced brain changes may be the reason weigh control is so hard. J of Clin Invest. 2012;122(1):153-162.

3. McNay D, et al. Remodeling of the arcuate nucleus energy-balance circuit is inhibited in mice. J Clin Invest. 2012;122(1):142-152

4. Fernandez et al. Study connects workplace turmoil, stress and obesity. Science Daily, March 24, 2010.

5. Cordain L, Friel S. Paleo Diet for Athletes. 2005, Rodale, USA.

6. Leproult R, Copinschi G, Buxton O, et al. Sleep loss results in an elevation of cortisol levels the next evening, Sleep. 1997;20:865-870.

7. Van Cauter, E. et al. Metabolic consequences of sleep and sleep loss. Sleep Med. 2008 Sep;9 Suppl 1:S23-8.

8. Uno H et al. Neurotoxicity of glucocorticoids in the primate brain. Horm Behav 28 (4):336-48.

9. Gillespie C., Nemeroff C. Hypercortisolemia and depression. Psychosom Med 67 Suppl 1:S26-28. Review.

10. Manetti L et al. Usefulness of salivary cortisol in the diagnosis of hyper-cortisolism: comparison with serum and urinary cortisol. 2013. Eur J Endocrinol 168(3):315-21

11. Cadore E et al. Correlations between serum and salivary hormonal concentrations in response to resistance exercise. J Sports Sci. 2008 Aug;26(10):1067-72.

12. Thayer JF, Sternberg E. Beyond heart rate variability: vagal regulation of allostatic systems. Ann NY Acad Sci 2006 Nov;1088:361-72.

13. Hellard P et al. Modeling the association between HR variability and illness in elite swimmers. Med Sci Sports Exerc. 2011 Jun;43(6):1063-7

14. Antonio, J et al. Essentials of Sports Nutrition and Supplements. Humana Press. New York, NY.

15. Peters Em. Vitamin C supplementation attenuates the increases in circulating cortisol, adrenaline and anti-inflammatory polypeptides following ultrama-rathon running. Int J Sports Med. 2001 Oct; 22(7):537-43.

16. Turakitwanakan W et al. Effects of mindfulness meditation on serum cortisol of medical students. J Med Assoc Thai 2013 Jan;96 Suppl 1:S90-5

17. Wurtzen H et al. Mindfulness significantly reduces self-reported levels of anxiety and depression: results of a randomised controlled trial among 336 Danish women treated for stage I-III breast cancer. Eur J Cancer 2013 Apr;49(6):1365-73.

18. DiPerri R. et al. A multicenter trial to evaluate the efficacy and tolerability of alpha-glycerylphosphorylcholine versus cytosine diphosphocholine in patients with vascular dementia. J Int Med Res. 1991. Jul-Aug;19(4):330-41.

19. Starks et al. The effects of phosphatidylserine on endocrine response to moderate intensity exercise. J Int Soc Sports Nutr 2008 Jul 28;5:11

20. Kingsley M. Effects of phosphatidylserine supplementation on exercising humans. Sports Med. 2006;36(8):657-69.

21. Chevalier A. Encyclopedia of Medicinal Plants. New York: DK Publishing, 1996

22. Mills S, Bone K. Principles and Practice of Phytotherapy. Edinburgh:Churchill Livingstone, 2000.

23. Bhattacharya SK et al. Anxiolytic-antidepressant activity of Withania somnifera glycowithanolides: an experimental study. Phytomedicine 2000 Dec; 7(6): 463-9.

Chapter 9
1. Guyton, A. Hall, J. Textbook of Medial Physiology, 10th Ed. Guyton Physiology. 2010

2. Feinamnn RD, Fine EJ. "A calorie is a calorie?" violates the second law of thermodynamics. Nutr J 2004;3:9.

3. Cameron JD et al. Increased meal frequency does not promote greater weight loss in subjects who were prescribed an 8-week equi-energetic energy-restricted diet. Br J Nutr 2010 Apr;103(8):1098-101

4. Munsters MJ, Saris WH. Effects of meal frequency on metabolic profiles and substrate partitioning in lean healthy males. PLos One 2012;7(6):e38632. Epub 2012 Jun 13

5. Smeets A, Westerterp-Plantegna M. Acute effects on metabolism and appetite profile of one meal difference in the lower range of meal frequency. Br J Nutr. 2008 Jun;99(6):1361-21.

6.   Arciero PJ, et al. Increased protein intake and meal frequency reduces abdominal fat during energy balance and energy deficit. Obesity (Silver Springs) 2013, 21:1357-1366.

7.   Johnson F, Wardle J. The association between weight loss and engagement with a web-based food and exercise diary in a commercial weight loss programme: a retrospective analysis. Int J Behav Nutr Phys Act. 2011 Aug 2;8:83

8.   Bahr R, et al. "Effect of exercise on recovery changes in plasma levels of FFA, glycerol, glucose and catecholamines". *Acta Physiologica Scandinavica* 143 (1): 105–15.

9.   Jackson AS, Pollock ML. Practical assessment of body composition. Phys Sports Med 1985;13:76-90.

10.   Lean et al. Waist circumference as a measure for indicating the need for weight management BMJ 1995 vol 311 p158-161.

11.   Paoli et al. Effect of ketogenic Mediterranean diet with phytoextracts and low carbohydrates/high-protein meals on weight, cardiovascular risk factors, body composition and diet compliance in Italian council employees. Nutr J 2011 Oct 12;10:112.

12.   Antonio, J et al. Essentials of Sports Nutrition and Supplements. Humana Press. New York, NY.

13.   Heilbronn LK et al. Energy restriction and weight loss on very low-fat diets reduce C-reacctive protein concentrations in obese, healthy women. Arterioscler Thromb Vasc Biol 2001;21:968-970.

14.   Volek JS et al. Comparison of energy restricted very low carbohydrate and low-fat diets on weight loss and body composition in overweight men and women. Nutr Metab (Lond) 2004;1-13.

15.   Brehm BJ et al. A randomized trial comparing a very low carbohydrate diet and a calorie restricted low fat diet on body weight and cardiovascular risk factors in healthy women. J clin Endocrinol Metab 2003;88:1617-1623.

16.   Scott CB. The effect of time under-tension and weight lifting cadence on aerobic, anaerobic, and recovery energy expenditures: 3 submaximal sets. Appl Physiol Nutr Metab. 2012 Apr;37(2):252-6

Chapter 10

1. Kilic M et al The effect of exhaustion exercise on thyroid hormones and testosterone levels of elite athletes receiving oral zinc. Neuro Endocrinol Lett. 2006 Feb-Apr;27(1-2):247-52

2. Hickson RC et al. Successive time courses of strength development and steroid hormone responses to heavy-resistance training. J Appl Physiol 1994;76:663-670.

3. Kraemer et al. Acute hormonal responses in elite junior weightlifeters. Int J Sports Med 1992;13:103-109

4. Fahey T et al. Serum testosterone, body composition, and strength of young adults. Med Sci Sports Exerc 1976;8:31-34.

5. Hansen et al. The effect of short-term strength training on human skeletal muscle: the importance of physiologically elevated hormone levels. Scand Med Sci Sport 2001;11:347-354.

6. Hakkinen et al. Acute hormonal responses to two different fatiguing heavy-resistance protocols in male athletes. J Appl Physiol 1993;74:882-887.

7. Rasstad T, et al. Hormonal response to high and moderate intensity strength exercise. Eur J Appl Physiol 2000:82:121-128

8. Kraemer et al. The effects of L-carnitine L-tartrate supplementation on hormonal responses to resistance exercise and recovery. J Strength Cond Res 2003;17:455-462

9. Stark et al. Protein timing and its effects on muscular hypertrophy and strength in individuals engaged in weight-training Journal of the International Society of Sports Nutrition 2012, 9:54

10. Frankenfield D, et al. Comparison of predictive equations for resting metabolic rate in healthy nonobese and obese adults: a systematic review. J Am Diet Assoc. 2005 May;105(5):775-89

11. Burd NA et al. Greater stimulation of myofibrillar protein synthesis with ingestion of whey protein isolate v. micellar casein at rest and after resistance exercise in elderly men. Br J Nutr. 2012 Sep 28;108(6):958-62.

12. Hoffman J, Falvo M: Protein—which is best? J Sports Sci Med 2004, 3:118–130.

13. Volek et al. testosterone and cortisol in relationship to dietary nutrients and resistance training exercise. J Appl Physiol 1997;8:49-54

14. Stellingwerff T et al. Nutrition for power sports: middle-distance running, track cycling, rowing, canoeing/kayaking, and swimming. J Sports Sci. 2011;29 Suppl 1:S79-89. Epub 2011 Jul 28.

15. Coffey VG et al. Nutrient provision increases signalling and protein synthesis in human skeletal muscle after repeated sprints. Eur J Appl Physiol. 2011 Jul;111(7):1473-83.

16. Tipton et al. Timing amino-acid carbohydrate ingestion alters anabolic response of muscle to resistance exercise. Am J Physiol Endocrinol Metab 281:E197-E206, 2001.

17. Ivy J. Muscle glycogen synthesis before and after exercise. Sports Med 1991; 11:6-11.

18. Beelen M et al. Protein coingestion stimulates muscle protein synthesis during resistance-type exercise. Am J Physiol Endocrinol Metab 2008 Jul;295(1):E70-7.

19. Baty JJ et al. The effect of a carbohydrate and protein supplement on resistance exercise performance, hormonal response, and muscle damage. J Strength Cond Res 2007 May;21(2):321-9

20. Samadi A et al. Effect of various ratios of carbohydrate-protein supplementation on resistance exercise-induced muscle damage. . J Sports Med Phys Fitness. 2012 Apr;52(2):151-7.

21. Blom P et al. Effects of different post-exercise sugar diets on the rate of muscle glycogen synthesis. Med Sci Sports Exerc 1987;19:491-496.

22. Kopman R et al. Ingestion of a protein hydrolysate is accompanied by an accelerated in vivo digestion and absorption rate when compared with its intact protein. Am J Clin Nutr. 2009 Jul;90(1):106-15

23. Kraemer WJ. Hormonal mechanisms related to the expression of muscular strength and power. Strength and Power in Sport. Cambridge, MA:Blackwell Scientific, 1992,64-76.

24. Elliot T, Cree M, Sanford A, Wolfe R, Tipton K: Milk ingestion stimulates net muscle protein synthesis following resistance exercise. Med Sci Sports Exerc 2006, 38(4):667–674.

25. Antonio, J et al. Essentials of Sports Nutrition and Supplements. Humana Press. New York, NY

26. Areta, J. L. (2013). "Timing and distribution of protein ingestion during prolonged recovery from resistance exercise alters myofibrillar protein synthesis." The Journal of physiology 591: 2319-2331.

27. Willoughby DS, Rosene JM. Effects of oral creatine and resistance training on myogenic regulatory factor expression. Med Sci Sports Exerc. 2003 Jun;35(6):923-9.

28. Buford TW et al. International Society of Sports Nutrition position stand: creatine supplementation and exercise. J Int Soc Sports Nutr 2007 Aug 30; 4:6 2007

29. Volek J, Rawson E. Nutrition. Scientific basis and practical aspects of creatine supplementation for athletes. 2004 Jul-Aug;20(7-8):609-14

ABOUT THE AUTHOR

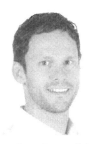 Dr. Marc Bubbs, ND, CSCS is a board-certified Naturopathic Doctor, Strength Coach, Speaker, Blogger, and Sports Nutrition Lead for the Canadian Men's Olympic Basketball Team. He has been working with athletes, active people, and those striving to improve their health for over a decade and is passionate that diet, exercise, and lifestyle factors are the foundation for better health and performance. Dr. Bubbs practices in Toronto, Canada and speaks across North America.

DrBubbs.com
PaleoProjectBook.com

📷 @DrBubbs

🐦 @DrBubbs

f DrBubbs